# WOMEN IN MEDICINE

## MEDICINE

### THIRD EDITION

**Springer**
*New York*
*Berlin*
*Heidelberg*
*Barcelona*
*Hong Kong*
*London*
*Milan*
*Paris*
*Singapore*
*Tokyo*

# WOMEN IN MEDICINE

THIRD EDITION

..............................................................................

## CAREER AND LIFE MANAGEMENT

MARJORIE A. BOWMAN, M.D., M.P.A.
*Professor and Founding Chair, Department of*
*Family Practice and Community Medicine*
*University of Pennsylvania Health Systems*
*Philadelphia, PA*

ERICA FRANK, M.D., M.P.H.
*Associate Professor and Vice Chair*
*Department of Family and Preventive Medicine*
*Emory University School of Medicine*
*Atlanta, GA*

DEBORAH I. ALLEN, M.D.
*Otis Bowen Professor and Director of*
*Bowen Research Center*
*Indiana University School of Medicine*
*Indianapolis, IN*

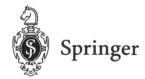 Springer

Marjorie A. Bowman, M.D., M.P.A.
Department of Family
  and Community Medicine
University of Pennsylvania Health Systems
2 Gates, 3400 Spruce Street
Philadelphia, PA 19104, USA
bowmanm@uphs.upenn.edu

Erica Frank, M.D., M.P.H.
Department of Family
  and Preventive Medicine
Emory University School of Medicine
69 Butler Street, SE
Atlanta, GA 30303, USA
efrank@learnlink.emory.edu

Deborah I. Allen, M.D.
Bowen Research Center
Indiana University School of Medicine
Long Hospital, Second Floor
1110 West Michigan Street
Indianapolis, IN 46202, USA
diallen@inpui.edu

Library of Congress Cataloging-in-Publication Data
Bowman, Marjorie A.
    Women in medicine : career and life management / Marjorie Bowman, Erica Frank,
    Deborah Allen.—3rd ed.
        p. cm.
    Rev. ed. of: Stress and women physicians / Marjorie A. Bowman, Deborah I. Allen. 2nd
ed. c1990.
    Includes bibliographical references and index.
    ISBN 0-387-95309-4 (alk. paper)
    1. Women physicians—Psychology.   2. Stress (Psychology)   3. Women
physicians—Mental health.   I. Frank, Erica.   II. Allen, Deborah I.   III. Bowman, Marjorie
A. Stress and women physicians.   IV. Title.
    [DNLM: 1. Physicians, Women—psychology.   2. Stress, Psychological.   W 21 B787w 2002]
R692 .B69 2002
610.69'52'082—dc21                                                          2001049253

Printed on acid-free paper.

Formerly *Stress and Women Physicians,* © 1990, 1988.

Production managed by Timothy Taylor; manufacturing supervised by Erica Bresler.
Composition by Impressions Book and Journal Services, Inc., Madison, WI.
Printed and bound by Edwards Brothers, Inc., Ann Arbor, MI.
Printed in the United States of America.

9  8  7  6  5  4  3  2  1

ISBN 0-387-95309-4                          SPIN 10841181

Springer-Verlag   New York  Berlin  Heidelberg
*A member of BertelsmannSpringer Science+Business Media GmbH*

# PREFACE

This is our third edition of an evolving book concerning the well-being of today's women physicians. Our experiences, a tremendous amount of new data, a changing medical milieu, and an additional major editor/author contribute to a substantial revision of our previous works.

The first and second editions of this book were entitled *Stress and Women Physicians* (Bowman MA, Allen DI, 1988, 1990, Springer-Verlag, NY). As we were planning for this third edition, we realized that though there are stresses in women physicians' lives, this was the wrong emphasis for the book. Of course, everyone, including women physicians, experiences stress. Like men physicians, women physicians have made considerable investments of time, emotion, and money to achieve their professional stature and have weighty professional responsibilities. Like other women, women physicians may have larger "second-shift" responsibilities at home than do many men. However, women physicians may also have disproportionate joys and reliefs. Like other physicians, we have the privilege of jobs that improve and may even save others' lives, earn very good incomes, and are in an esteemed profession. And unlike most other women (and many men), because of our salaries we can afford to hire others to perform many dispensable tasks and can work fewer hours yet still earn enough to support our families.

This explanation and title change is not intended to negate the special and sometimes substantial stresses that women physicians may feel; indeed the major purpose of this book is to help women physicians cope with these stresses. However, we do not wish to support a nineteenth-century notion that if you educate women they somehow become otherwise bereft. As you will see in this book, there is substantial evidence that women physicians usually thrive; our aim is to make that thriving condition even more common!

The woman who chooses medicine as a career faces many challenges. Women have consistently been shown to be equally competent to men physicians. However, the numbers of women in the field has increased dramatically in recent years without the achievement of equality with men at many levels—pay, academic advancement, and power. With an authority structure dominated by men, the norms in medicine are long working hours and the perception that a career as a physician is more important than family ties or time.

Because of their increased numbers, women physicians may feel less isolated and have more role models. Although this will provide a positive influence, it will not remove the continued need for decision making and priority setting concerning personal life and career, an issue men also face, but for which they may have fewer expectations for participation in home life and child-rearing.

As long as there are women physicians, there will be women's issues. Particular needs will change with time, external events, and individual women themselves. This book is intended as a picture of today's women physicians, as well as thought-provoking resource on dealing with the joys and challenges of being a woman physician in the new millenium.

The third edition is a monument to the current intense interest in the issues of women physicians. The amount of research and commentary that has been written about women physicians in the last few years has been tremendous, expanding our understanding of the role of women in medicine. This edition includes much information from a major new project called the Women Physicians' Health Study, which is described in more detail in the introduction. We have also added additional authors and new chapters on disabilities, and minority and older women physicians. Because of advancing laws and legal cases, information on sexual harassment and discrimination have been significantly updated.

We hope this book will be useful to all women physicians and to interested others, and will provide as much of a learning experience for its readers as it has for its authors.

Marjorie A. Bowman
Philadelphia, PA

Erica Frank
Atlanta, GA

Deborah I. Allen
Indianapolis, IN

# ACKNOWLEDGMENTS

I would like to thank:

- Jamillah Hoy for her always pleasant library research support.
- Todd Bracey for working with my computer frequently, often urgently, when I was in a panic.
- My husband, my stepchildren, and my children for loving me, teaching me much about life, accepting my love, and supporting me . . . even if I write books.
- My mother and my now-deceased father for being great forces and support in my life.
- Esther Gumpert, our editor, for believing in us, encouraging us, and steadfastly working with us, even in her retirement.
- The many women physicians, including my coauthors, who have shared their stories, challenges, and triumphs with me and to whom I look for my inspiration.

Marjorie A. Bowman, M.D., M.P.A.

I would like to acknowledge my two partners: Dorothy Fitzmaurice, my partner at work, and Randall White, my partner at home. Little of importance would happen in either place without their thoughtful and firm guidance and their enormous dedication to the tasks we have undertaken together. I would also like to acknowledge Lisa Elon, who is responsible for producing data for the Women's Physicians' Health Study (WPHS) that is as impressively solid as she is, and the brilliant and delightful health providers-in-training who have also worked on WPHS. I'd also like to thank my Chairman, Larry Lutz, for believing in me and consistently acting on that belief. I would also like to thank the generous responders to WPHS and the authors and readers of this book for their time and commitment. Finally, I want to thank my parents, Ulrich and Ruth Frank, for the unsurpassed opportunities they gave me, and my in-laws, Jim and Lucia Cowan, for the opportunities they are giving my wonderful son, Ridge Frank-White.

Erica Frank, M.D., M.P.H.

I would like to thank my family. My two children remain a constant joy. They have helped me put many of my thoughts from this book into action. They continue to be a constant support for their mother. I would also like to thank my parents, Ted and Louise Allen. From them I have learned the value of education and continued learning. And finally I would like to thank all the women physicians who have been the inspiration for this book.

Deborah I. Allen, M.D.

# ABOUT THE EDITORS

**Marjorie A. Bowman, M.D., M.P.A.,** is a professor and founding chair, Department of Family Practice and Community Medicine, University of Pennsylvania Health System, Philadelphia, Pennsylvania. Previously, she was a professor and chair of the Department of Family and Community Medicine at Bowman Gray School of Medicine, Wake Forest University, and she has been president of the Society of Teachers of Family Medicine, the Society of Teachers of Family Medicine Foundation, and the American Board of Family Practice. She is a member of the Institute of Medicine, and she was the youngest woman physician (and pregnant) at the time of her induction to this prestigious group. She has published many medical articles and books and was the founding editor of the *Archives of Family Medicine*. Her medical degree is from Jefferson Medical College, and her family practice residency was at Duke University. She is board certified in both family practice and preventive medicine. She is married and has three stepchildren (in college or out on their own) and two children in the home. Her husband is an academic radiologist. Her mother shares their home.

**Erica Frank, M.D., M.P.H.,** is a tenured associate professor at Emory University and vice chair of the Department of Family and Preventive Medicine. She completed a residency (Yale, 1990) and fellowship (Stanford, 1993) in preventive medicine, and is the former editor of the journal *Preventive Medicine* (1994–1999). She is the principal investigator of the Women Physicians' Health Study (which is described in considerable detail in this book) and the "Healthy Doc—Healthy Patient" project (an 18–medical school project to cultivate healthy personal habits among physicians so that they will become more avid preventionists). Among other volunteer roles, she serves on the national boards of the American College of Preventive Medicine and Physicians for Social Responsibility. She is married to a psychiatrist/environmental activist, and they have a 5-year-old son. She lives in co-housing in Atlanta and in an energy-independent home in a corner of the Southern Nantahala Wilderness.

**Deborah I. Allen, M.D.,** is currently the Otis Bowen Professor and director of the Bowen Research Center at Indiana University School of Medicine, Indiana University, Indianapolis, Indiana. Previously she was the chair of the Department of Family Medicine from 1989 to 1998. Dr. Allen is the past president of the American Board of Family Practice. She is also a delegate to the American Medical Association from the American Academy of Family Physicians. Her medical degree is from Indiana University School of Medicine, and her family practice residency was at Methodist Hospital in Indianapolis. She is board certified in family medicine. Dr. Allen is divorced and has two sons, ages 16 and 12.

# CONTENTS

# CONTRIBUTORS

**Vignette Contributors**

Tamara Bavendam, M.D.: Associate Professor of Surgery/Urology; Director, Center for Women's Health at MCP, MCP Hahnemann University, Philadelphia, PA.

Janet Bickel: Experienced Speaker/Writer on women in medicine issues; Association of American Medical Colleges.

Catherine DeAngelis, M.D.: Editor, *JAMA*.

Nancy Dickey, M.D.: Family Physician, first and only (so far) woman president, American Medical Association, 1998–1999.

Phyllis Kopriva: Director, Women and Minority Services, American Medical Association.

Mary LaPlante, M.D.: Young Physicians' Section Representative to the American Medical Association Women Physicians' Congress.

Diane Shrier, M.D.: Clinical Professor of Psychiatry and Pediatrics, George Washington University Medical Center, Washington, DC.

Lydia Shrier, M.D.: Instructor, Pediatrics, Harvard Medical School; Assistant in Medicine, Division of Adolescent/Young Adult Medicine, Children's Hospital, Boston (daughter of Dr. Diane Shrier).

**Chapter Contributors**

Jada Bussey-Jones, M.D.: Senior Associate, Department of Internal Medicine, Emory University School of Medicine, Atlanta, GA.

Alicia Conill, M.D.: Clinical Professor of Medicine, University of
    Pennsylvania, Philadelphia, PA
Giselle Corbie-Smith, M.D.: Assistant Professor of Medicine, University of
    North Carolina School of Medicine, Chapel Hill, NC
Meredith Mitchell: Medical Student, Medical University of South Carolina,
    Charleston, SC.

# Introduction: The Women Physicians' Health Study

Dr. Erica Frank is the Principal Investigator for the Women Physicians' Health Study (WPHS). This is a survey study of 10,000 women physicians, funded primarily by the American Heart Association, the American Medical Association Foundation and the Emory Medical Care Foundation. The sample was stratified, evenly divided between women randomly selected from each of the last four decades' graduating classes. It includes women who are practicing, inactive, and retired. The survey asks questions about both professional and personal lives, including sociodemographic and psychosocial characteristics, health behaviors, health status, and counseling practices. The first survey was sent in September 1993, and the enrollment was closed in October 1994. The response rate was 59% of the eligible physicians ($N = 4,501$). A partial bibliogaphy from WPHS is included in the back of this book; an updated bibliography can be found at the website for WPHS, http://med.emory.edu/WPHS/.

## CHAPTER 1

# HISTORICAL CONTEXT

Marjorie A. Bowman

Women have practiced medicine for many centuries. In ancient Egypt there were many women students and women professors in the medical schools and, in about 1500 B.C., both Moses and his wife were students of medicine (Turner 1981). There has also been a long history of discrimination against women in medicine, recorded at least as early as 1421, when a petition was presented to King Henry V to prevent women from practicing medicine (Heins 1979). The first formal degree awarded to a woman is said to have been to Constanza Collenda in 1431 (Nadelson 1983).

Before the nineteenth century, the most common type of health care giver was the female midwife; labor and delivery were considered too "dirty and debasing" for men (Fidell 1980). It was not until the nineteenth century that men began entering obstetrics/gynecology in large numbers, and discrimination against women as physicians became powerful, vocal, and open, often on the basis of economic competition. An 1848 textbook on obstetrics, for example, stated that a woman's head was too small for intellect, but just "big enough for love" (Shyrock 1966). Thus, it said, women should not practice medicine. Medical schools would not admit women. Harvard Medical School was going to admit a woman, Harriet Hunt, in 1850 but did not do so after the male student body protested strongly (Walsh 1977). In spite of this initial rejection, Dr. Hunt is credited with being the first woman to successfully practice medicine in the United States, beginning in 1835 (Walsh 1977), and became known as the "mother of the American woman physician" (Abram 1985).

In spite of the admission of the first woman to a "regular" medical school, Elizabeth Blackwell to Geneva Medical College in 1847, which many thought to be an accident (Abram 1985), there continued to be a lack of opportunity for women in medical schools. As a result, three medical schools specifically for women were opened by 1864: in Boston, Philadelphia, and Cincinnati (Walsh 1977). The first black woman physician, Rebecca Lee, graduated in 1864 from the New England Female Medical College in Boston (Abram 1985). Medical societies, however, continued to refuse admission to women, and it was exceptionally difficult for women to receive an academic appointment outside a women's medical school. In 1868, Howard University Medical School was chartered and supported by the government to train black physicians (Abram 1985). By 1870, the percentage of women physicians in the United States was only 0.8% (Heins 1979), very few of whom were minorities.

The long struggles of women to be accepted as medical students, interns, and physicians in the late 1800s is well researched and recorded in three books: *Doctors Wanted: No Women Need Apply* (Walsh 1977), *Send Us a Lady Physician: Women Doctors in American 1835–1920* (Abram 1985), and *Sympathy and Science: Women Physicians in American Medicine* (Morantz-Sanchez 1985).

Some success was achieved when combined fund raising efforts, and a particularly large sum of money from one woman, created a $500,000 endowment at Johns Hopkins University in return for the equal admission of men and women, beginning in 1893. In spite of this, only 16% of the students were women in 1893–94 and 7% in 1907–08. However, gains were made; by 1900, women constituted 18.2% of all physicians in Boston, and 42% of the graduating class from Tufts University. In the United States at that time, 6% of all physicians were women (Abram 1985).

*More men than women feel that women have made a lot of progress at work, as customers, and in the media's portrayal of them (Hunt AR. Major progress, inequities cross three generations. Wall Street Journal, Thursday, June 22, 2000, page A9).*

Unfortunately, the success women physicians gained by 1900 was temporary. For a variety of reasons, a number of the medical colleges created for women either merged with male schools or closed. The percentage of women physicians declined to 4.4% of physicians by 1940, and did not again reach over 6% until 1950, after the influx of women medical students during the war years (Walsh 1977). Even in the mid-1970s, discrimination against women on the part of some medical schools was overt in the listing of their medical school admission requirements (Walsh 1977).

> "Hard study killed sexual desire in women. It took away their beauty, brought on hysteria, neurasthenia, dyspepsia, stygmatism, and dysmenorrhea." Educated women could "not bear children with ease because study arrested the development of the pelvis."
>     Dr. Van Dyk, President of the Oregon State Medical Society, 1905 (Bullough 1973).

There was a continual slow rise in the numbers of women in medicine in the United States from the early 1900s until another major surge in numbers started during the 1970s. In 1970–71, the percentage of women in medical schools was 8.9%, reaching 43% in 1997–98 (Bickel et al 1998). The percentage of women physician overall had advanced to 22% by the end of 1997 (AMA 1999).

Women have, in spite of their low numbers as physicians, been the majority of workers in the health care sector [about 85% (Brown 1975)], although the minority in leadership positions. Women will have to do more than increase their numbers to have an impact at the leadership level.

Thus, women represent a growing minority of the physicians in the United States. Many battles have been fought to achieve the current standing for women, but substantial inequality persists.

## CHAPTER 2

# THE STRESS
# OF OUR PROFESSION

DEBORAH I. ALLEN AND MARJORIE A. BOWMAN

Stress reactions are probably genetically ingrained from our early ancestry. The "fight or flight" response served our ancestors well. When a saber-toothed tiger approached, the sympathetic nervous system reacted automatically. The heart rate increased along with blood pressure. Breathing became shallow, and muscles tensed for action. Blood flow to the extremities decreased and fingers and feet became colder. In modern society these automatic responses have lost their evolutionary advantage. Although there are no longer saber-toothed tigers, the prehistoric stress response remains. It is estimated that approximately $75 billion a year is lost on illness and absenteeism related to stress in the United States (Walis 1983).

## RESEARCH ON STRESS

The "father of stress" is Dr. Hans Selye (1976), who defined stress as the non-specific response of the body to any change or demand. This means any change, positive or negative, can induce stress. Stress can also be additive. The seemingly minor hassles of everyday life can add up to a substantial, chronic stress response. Selye examined brain tissue after physical stress and found that the level of norepinephrine dropped 20% and epinephrine dropped 40%. Stress also boosted the body's production of endorphins, which may be the body's natural mechanism for raising its threshold to pain. The alteration of the body's chemistry may potentiate the development of many diseases.

The stress response involves many body systems and includes such reactions as increased arousal and alertness; increased cognition, vigilance, and focused attention; suppression of feeding behavior; suppression of reproductive behavior; oxygen and nutrients directed to the central nervous system and the stressed body site; altered cardiovascular tone; increased blood pressure and heart rate; increased respiratory rate; increased gluconeogenesis and lipolysis; and inhibition of growth and reproductive systems (Chrousos and Gold 1992). The chronic activation of these systems can explain depression and other psychiatric disorders such as anorexia nervosa, panic anxiety, obsessive-compulsive disorder, excessive exercising, chronic alcoholism, malnutrition, and premenstrual syndrome (Chrousos and Gold 1992). As an example of this, in one study of 1,523 married professional and managerial employees of a major U.S. corporation, both occupational and domestic stresses were separately associated with depression (Phelan et al 1991).

Stress influences our immune responses (Glaser et al 1999). Glaser et al noted evidence of changes in cytokines as a result of stress hormones, less immune response to vaccines for stressed individuals, and greater susceptibility to the common cold when an individual is stressed. Genital herpes recurrences in women were associated with persistent stressors and high levels of anxiety but not short-term stressors or life change events (Cohen et al 1999).

Stress has also been linked to higher rates of heart disease and hypertension. For example, the more stressful the job, the higher the rise in blood pressure (Schnall 1998). Lack of control of the work environment is associated with heart disease (Johnson and Hall 1988; Karasek 1981 et al). La Rosa (1988) in her review of the literature concluded that perception of control over the job could be a greater risk factor for coronary heart disease than the level of other types of job distress. Mental stress testing can provoke myocardial ischemia (Krantz et al 2000). Anger, sadness, frustration, and tension all appear to be significant triggers of ischemia in patients with coronary artery disease (Krantz et al 2000). Conversely, better social support and better economic increases is associated with a better prognosis in cardiac patients (Krantz et al 2000). Depression after a heart attack is associated with increased mortality (Krantz et al 2000) and with the development of hypertension (Davidson et al 2000). Increases in the number of social interactions are associated with better cardiovascular health behaviors (Ford et al 2000).

## PHYSICIAN STRESS

Just as for nonphysicians, lack of control on the job is associated with psychiatric distress and job dissatisfaction, and the presence of social support at work is associated with more job satisfaction and less psychiatric distress for physicians (Johnson et al 1995). These two factors were far more important than the psychological or patient demands of the job, or the support resources (such as nursing staff or equipment) available. In another study of internal medicine residents, both adrenocorticotropic hormone (ACTH) and cortisol were increased after 24 hours on call, consistent with the experience being stressful (Coeck et al 1991).

## LACK OF CONTROL OF THE WORK ENVIRONMENT

Unfortunately, the exact traits that help us get through medical school and help advance our careers may actually add to our stress. Menninger (as cited by Lamberg 1999) found that many physicians seeking psychiatric help could not label or recognize their own feelings. Physicians are very intelligent and as a result use rationalization frequently as a coping mechanism. Doctors often come from family backgrounds in which there were high expectations. This creates an internal dialogue among many physicians that says, "If I work harder, I will be loved" (Lamberg 1999).

In a study of 4,500 physicians, 31% stated they would choose a different profession if they had to start over again (Neuwirth 1999). Work stress and poor control over their working environment left one-third of these physicians emotionally exhausted. Recent changes in the health care industry have compounded the problem. With the huge increase in managed health care organizations, physicians feel even more loss of control. Each organization has restrictive rules, endless paper forms, and directives that intrude on the doctor–patient relationship. With this loss of professional autonomy, it is easy to see why so many doctors are feeling significant stress. The rising incidence of malpractice claims also contribute to physician stress. Some physicians feel that each patient encounter is either a legal or financial threat.

## THE STRESS CURVE

The stress curve is a useful model for understanding stress and its effects on productivity (Chrousos and Gold 1992; Nixon 1976) (Figure 2-1). The $x$-axis plots the amount of stress or change a person is experiencing. Note there is no place on the graph where stress is nonexistent. The $y$-axis represents productivity or the individual's sense of well-being. The old adage that "stress is good for you" is true to a point. As stress increases so does productivity. After a certain critical point, fatigue intervenes and productivity starts decreasing. Further stress can cause exhaustion and burnout (Nixon 1976). The size of the stress graph can also vary according to a person's physical and mental state. After a night of call and missing a meal, a resident's ability to tolerate stress will be greatly decreased (Murphy 1981). The stress curve is obviously oversimplistic (King 1987), but it does provide a model for the potential impacts of stress on our lives and helps us to think about the potential, varying, impacts of stressful events on our lives.

FIGURE 2-1.
The stress curve

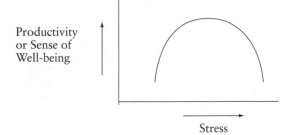

The amount of stress an individual can tolerate is influenced by many factors including the physiologic state and the adequacy of coping skills (Murphy 1981) (Figure 2-2).

## STRESS AND THE MEDICAL STUDENT

Likely all people have been, are, and will continue to be stressed. Although some aspects of medical training are uniquely stressful, many of the stresses experienced by medical students are similar to those of other students in graduate school (Gottheil 1969). The stresses also seem fairly stable over time. Compare the similar lists of factors that earned the highest mean stress scores in studies of medical students from 1975 and 1997 (Table 2-1).

Another unfortunate stress reaction is "medical student's disease." As students study an illness, they develop the symptoms of the illness (Woods 1966; Kellner 1986). Overall, medical students (in Ontario) reported lower overall

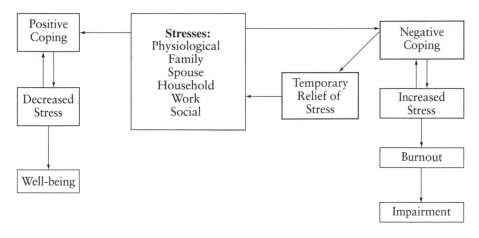

FIGURE 2-2.
The stress cycle

TABLE 2-1.
STRESS FACTORS FOR MEDICAL STUDENTS

| 1975[b] | 1997[a] |
|---------|---------|
| 1. Final examinations | 1. Large volume of material to know |
| 2. Fear of the inability to absorb the amount of course material | 2. Lack of time available to learn new material |
| 3. Fear of bad grades | 3. High self-expectations |
| 4. The huge number of hours needed for study | 4. Examinations/evaluations |
| 5. The limited recreational and social outlets | 5. Feelings of lack of competence |
| 6. The lack of sexual outlets | 6. Lack of money |
| 7. Feelings of loneliness | 7. Ambiguity of expectations |
| 8. Initial dissection of a cadaver | 8. Complexity of subject matter |

Source: [a]Adapted from Toews et al 1997 with permission.
[b]Adapted from Coburn and Jovaisis 1975 with permission.

general health perceptions and vitality than the U.S. general population, particularly during the clerkship years in which they were on call (Raj et al 2000). However, another report found health anxiety/hypochondriasis scores similar to those of law students, other students, and nonstudents (Kellner et al 1986).

## STRESS AND THE RESIDENT

The issue of resident stress rose to the forefront of national attention during the controversy surrounding the Libby Zion case in New York in 1988 (McCall 1988), in which a patient at New York Hospital–Cornell Medical Center died, possibly because of resident error due in part to overwork and lack of sleep. The resulting public fears about the quality of care given by overworked residents resulted in legislation regulating the work hours for residents in New York (Colford and McPhee 1989). Similar fears have caused the Accreditation Council on Graduate Medical Education to add into the general essentials for residency training specific guidelines for the amount of time residents can work. Various specialties have also defined the amount of time on call that is allowable in their Residency Review Committee guidelines.

Residents and other young health professionals experience stress from patient care responsibilities, concerns over personal development, and the changes in their lives (Cherniss 1980). However, there are some unique aspects of medical residency, many revolving around sleep deprivation and its effects. The most common stresses for residents are the following:

1. Sleep deprivation (Lurie 1989)
2. Large volume of material they must learn (Toews 1997)
3. Lack of personal time (Friedman et al 1973)

4. Applying for and repaying medical student loans (Blackwell 1986; Sandson 1985)
5. Moonlighting (McKegney 1989)
6. The demands of marriage (Myers 1988)

The medical education system is often described as "an abusive family system" (McKegney 1989). The system abounds with unrealistic expectations, denial, indirect communication patterns, and rigidity. Just like abusive parents who raise their children as they themselves were raised, each generation of medical educators tends to teach as it was taught. Acute sleep deprivation is associated with lower glucose tolerance, raised cortisol concentrations, and increased sympathetic nervous system activity (Spiegel et al 1999). Another study of residents before and after 36 hours of call found decreased sustained visual attention, speed and coding ability, and short-term recall; interestingly, hand–eye coordination improved (Rubin et al 1991).

## STRESS AND THE PRACTICING PHYSICIAN

After residents finish residency, they often believe that life will be less stressful. For some that may be true, but there are also new stressors, often revolving around having the ultimate responsibility for patients, increased financial risk, and responsibility for others. There are many emotional issues that are governed by strong cultural codes (McCue 1982). Residents move from being able to blame someone else (the system, the attending physician), to increasing uncertainty. Physicians enter the profession presuming they will cure patients and find that frequently they cannot control, let alone cure, the problems that occur in their practice. The following problems are the most stressful to practicing physicians:

1. Difficult patients (Spears 1981)
2. Sexual issues with patients (McCue 1982)
3. Death of patients
4. Hostile families of patients
5. Difficult diagnostic problems
6. Malpractice suits (Charles et al 1987)
7. Loss of autonomy
8. The business side of medicine

Negative coping mechanisms that do not address the underlying stress are as common in physicians as they are in the general public. One negative coping mechanism that appears to be used commonly by physicians is isolation (Haleran 1981). The doctor's energy is spent on work, with little left for personal relationships. This is compounded by the fact that doctors often receive positive reinforcement for spending extra time at the office. Physicians may also remove themselves from social activities. Unfortunately, this also cuts them off from valuable support networks.

## BURNOUT AND IMPAIRMENT

Burnout occurs in physicians when they no longer care about their work (Selder 1989). At this point they are usually numb. They have given of themselves until there is nothing left to give (Regelson 1989). A short step beyond burnout is impairment. Physicians are considered impaired when personal problems interfere with the quality of their medical care, personal life, or well-being. This dramatic outcome seems to be the end of a process that begins as much milder symptoms, with patterns that develop and proliferate many years before friends, colleagues, or the public become aware of or vocal about the doctor's problem. Physicians can also vacillate among impairment, improvement, and well-being, and then experience burnout and impairment again.

## FEMALE PHYSICIAN STRESSES

In one study, almost 65% of female family physicians felt overwhelmed at least once a week (Brown 1992). Women face unique stresses as physicians. Discrimination still exists in some schools and workplaces (Campbell 1973) (see Chapter 7). Sexual harassment continues to be present in the medical environment with a disproportionate amount occurring against females. Overall women seem to be more stressed than their male professional colleagues (Toews 1997). Females also complain of having less support from their employers and their families. Female physicians rely heavily on their spouse as their major source of support. The following are the most stressful situations for women physicians in descending order (Gross 1997):

1.  Conflict between career and personal life
2.  Sexual harassment
3.  Prejudice by patients, staff, and nurses

Women in medicine have been perceived as "violating" the existing group the same way any minority violates a majority. This can lead to stereotyping and prejudice from their male colleagues (Potter 1983). Overt discrimination occurs when teachers bait and tease women students (Campbell 1973). Women students may be stereotyped as "too masculine," "nonmothering," or "too pretty to be a medical student" (Cartwright 1987; Johnson 1988; Scott 1978). Until about 30 years ago, there were often no arrangements for female physicians to sleep in the hospital while on call (Campbell 1973). Women were forced to sleep wherever they could find an empty bed. Some locker rooms to this day continue to be labeled "doctors" and "nurses." Complaints about such issues are often viewed as less than "sisterly."

Although women have come a long way in medicine, female medical students still lack many role models in the higher academic ranks such as full professors and department chairs. Furthermore, any one woman can represent only one arrangement of many possible lifestyles (Nadelson and Notman 1972). In one study, 19% of the women in practice felt that their career development was inhibited by the lack of same-sex role models (Cohen et al 1988), an encouragingly low percentage. The presence of women who have "made it," who have successfully dealt with being a woman physician and who are confident, secure, and professional, creates a lasting impression and provides a basis for the individual's own sense of self-worth.

So what is a woman physician to do? Chapter 3 addresses this question.

# STRESS PREVENTION AND MANAGEMENT

DEBORAH I. ALLEN AND MARJORIE A. BOWMAN

Life is stressful—a condition that can be compounded for physicians. One solution to the dilemma of managing stress lies in prevention. Some proponents of this method have suggested prescreening medical school applicants for their ability to handle stress and teaching values clarification during medical school (Spears 1981). Others have suggested making support groups, stress management techniques, and methods for early identification of problems during medical training a part of every medical school (Gerber 1983; Hoferik 1981).

Dealing with the problems and stresses of being a physician is not easy. There continues to be a macho attitude underlying the commonly held view that internships and residencies should be trials by ordeal. Until this basic underlying attitude changes, it will be difficult to address the stresses of medical training. In the meantime, courses or workshops in primary prevention techniques such as stress recognition, stress management, and interpersonal skills could be highly beneficial for medical students, residents, and, in the long run, physicians.

The literature is long on identifying the problems of physician stress and impairment but short on adequate solutions (Spears 1981). Although about one in five Fortune 500 companies has developed some sort of stress management program for their top-level executives (Walis 1983), this practice has not been widely adopted by medical schools.

There is no single approach to stress management that is right for everyone; as the response to stress varies widely, so does the treatment. However, the same advice that physicians give patients for identifying stress and learning to respond adaptively is applicable to physicians themselves (Spears 1981): one person may need a prescription for exercise and time off, whereas another may need psychotherapy.

## DEALING WITH STRESS

The current lay literature abounds with help on dealing with the stresses of life. In many ways the answers for physicians are the same. Several recent studies have helped delineate the coping strategies of physicians who seem to remain happier and more contented in their lives than most of their counterparts. Some patterns for coping among these individuals are (Post 1997):

1. Stress monitoring: Physicians who are constantly aware of their feelings were able to identify when they are overly stressed.
2. Action: This is a specific planned activity to counter the identified stress.
3. A positive perspective: Successful physicians were always looking for the positive aspects of their situations.
4. Support: Healthy doctors had a full range of support including family, friends, and colleagues.
5. Self-care: All of the physicians who were successful took time to care for their own emotional and physical needs.
6. Spiritual life: The contented doctors in this study all had a spiritual side of their life that they nurtured.

Successful women physicians use these coping strategies. Other factors that correlate with better mental health and well-being in women physicians are having well-educated parents and certain personality characteristics, such as being less hostile, cynical, and angry, and more open-minded, fluid, and optimistic (Cartwright 1987). There are other personality characteristics that are effective in coping for women physicians (McLean 1982; Wallis 1983):

1. A sense of being in control of one's life
2. The ability to change and be flexible
3. Optimism—the attitude that there is hope in most circumstances
4. A deep commitment to some goal or belief

Barnett (1987) described a similar concept called, "hardiness," which combines commitment (to something one is doing), control (actions and belief that one can influence outcome), and challenge (belief that change is normative).

## RECOGNITION OF STRESS

It may be difficult for professionals to recognize and especially to admit that stress may be affecting them and their health. But by watching for the effects of stress, it is possible to take early corrective action to prevent impairment. The signs of stress are classic but vary from person to person. Thus, each individual needs to know her/his own stress cures. For example, one person's stress may cause headaches, a stiff neck, or a nagging backache. Another person may become irritable and intolerant of even minor disturbances by other people and start yelling at others without cause. The heart rate usually increases with acute stress, and a feeling of exhaustion even after a good night's sleep is common. Recognizing these as signs of stress is the first step in combating it (Jasmine and Hill 1981).

Using a stress questionnaire is another method for recognition. A popular one, the Holmes-Rahle Social Readjustment, scale was created by psychiatrists Thomas Holmes and Richard Rahle (1976) to rate the impact of life events as stressors. The psychiatrists' research showed that in a sample of 88 young physicians, those with a scale score of 300 or more had a 70% chance of suffering from ulcers, psychiatric disturbances, broken bones, or other health problems within the ensuing two years. Those who scored under 200 had only a 37% chance of such illness. The Holmes-Rahle Social Readjustment Rating Scale has proven to be an effective prognosticator of stress-related illnesses (Walis 1983). Reviewing this scale and its indicators of stress can be useful for the physician.

Another method of stress recognition is identification of one's own personality characteristics that have been associated with a likelihood of increased stress. The scale, Personal Risk Factors for Stress for Women Physicians (Table 3-1), provides an assessment of the aspects of one's personality that could lead

TABLE 3-I.
PERSONAL RISK ANALYSIS FOR STRESS FOR WOMEN PHYSICIANS

|  | Yes | No |
| --- | --- | --- |
| 1. Is maintaining your superwoman image important? |  |  |
| 2. Do you let your practice take control of your life? |  |  |
| 3. Are your family's and patients' needs more important than your own? |  |  |
| 4. Do you feel overloaded all the time? |  |  |
| 5. Do you blame others for your problems? |  |  |
| 6. Is it hard for you to delegate work at home and at the office? |  |  |
| 7. Do you find it difficult to change behaviors? |  |  |
| 8. Are you waiting for someone else to help reduce your stress? |  |  |
| 9. Do you receive positive feedback on the "mother" role? |  |  |
| 10. Do you continually strive to achieve? |  |  |
| 11. Are you considered too intense? |  |  |
| 12. Do you lack support from friends and family? |  |  |

Count the number of yes responses:

_____  0–3   Minimal risk
_____  4–8   Moderate risk
_____  9–12  Significant risk

to stress. Factors indicating a high likelihood should give you pause for reflection on their importance in your life.

The type of coping style is also important. Blake and Vandiver (1988) found that an active-cognitive style of coping was positively and avoidance-coping was negatively associated with health status. Active-cognitive coping included such things as trying to see the positive side, trying to step back from the situation and be more objective, praying for guidance or strength, taking things one step at a time, considering several alternatives for handling problems, and drawing on past experiences (recognition of dealing with a similar situation before). Attempting to block stress-producing beliefs through positive self-statements (such as those based on the above active-cognitive coping style) and positive imagery is called stress inoculation (King 1987).

## BASIC STRESS REDUCING TECHNIQUES

There has been a lot written about management of stress, but most of the basic techniques appear to be simply common sense (Jamine and Hill 1981; King 1987; Loehr 1997; Murphy 1981; Walis 1983):

1. Keep your weight at its ideal level.
2. Don't smoke.
3. Don't use caffeine.
4. Exercise regularly.
5. Get enough sleep.
6. Take time out for yourself regularly and use relaxation techniques.
7. Participate in enjoyable activities outside of work.
8. Avoid unnecessary stressful situations.
9. Plan in advance to make a known situation less stressful. Plan your possible responses.
10. Decide if an issue is worth the stress. Changed expectations can greatly reduce stress.
11. Try to find humor in your daily activities. Most of us need to lighten up a bit.

## CAREER PATTERNS

One common solution to role strain for women physicians has been to back off from ambition. But many play wonderwoman, and hang on to all of the old domestic roles while pursuing a career full blast. The negative affects of this can be extreme role strain, fatigue, anxiety, and resentment about having too much work to do and never enough time (Dowling 1981). There are three basic options in terms of career patterns as described by Rapoport and

Rapoport (1971) for women faced with the roles of mother, wife, and physician:

1. Conventional—The woman drops her career when she marries or after childbearing and concentrates on being a housewife and mother with no intention of returning to work. This is unusual for female physicians.
2. Interrupted—The woman diminishes her work for a period of time when her children are young with all intentions of returning to work. A few pilot projects for retraining inactive physicians have been successful in permitting women to reenter active medical practice (Brown 1969; Wineberg 1972).
3. Continuous—The woman interrupts her career only minimally or not at all for childbearing.

Each of these is a viable option with its own pros and cons depending on an individual's situation. Cartwright (1987) has described a "role montage," which represents the complexities of changing patterns and priorities over the lifetime of a woman's career development and the changing nature of the demands of the roles over time.

There has been little support for the multiple roles of women in medicine. If the woman physician decides to combine motherhood and marriage with medicine, she will profit from adopting the philosophy that these roles are indeed compatible and simultaneously her right. Symonds (1979) claims that some women do not believe they are entitled to achieve—a significant inhibitor to the achievement in itself. She has found that some women have serious difficulties nurturing their own inner growth and development. Younger women appear to be developing a healthier sense of entitlement to all that life can offer; it is hoped that this trend will continue to grow as more women enter medicine.

## TECHNIQUES FOR REDUCING ROLE STRAIN

Here are several techniques:

1. Role cycling—allowing yourself to give higher priority to one or another role at different times.
2. Subjective rationalization—attributing one's actions to rational and creditable motives regardless of the unconscious reasons; for example, believing that it is not the quantity of time you spend with your children, but the quality of time that is important to their well-being.
3. Changed expectations—learning to develop a flexible attitude toward daily problems; for example, teaching children to be more self-reliant and independent, allowing others to help in ways that may suit them better than you or letting the housework go.
4. Decreased confrontation with societal norms—avoiding situations that highlight differences with others. For example, dual-career couples can

choose friends with similar backgrounds, thus reducing conflict (Rapoport and Rapoport 1971). Alternatively, one can increase one's comfort level with ways in which one differs from societal norms.

5. Creative child care—reducing stress and role strain when the parents are comfortable with the child care arrangements.

6. Hire help!—decreasing role strain by hiring help, probably several kinds: someone to help take care of the children, someone to mow the lawn and landscape the yard, someone to fix the car, someone to do the housework, someone to deliver the groceries, and someone to select and purchase clothes for you. Hiring costs money, but health and happiness are more important. It has been said that what all women physicians need is a good wife!

7. Stay close—concentrating your life—work, home, schools, and major social supports—in a small geographic area.

## TIME MANAGEMENT

Stress is unavoidable. You will need to identify the personal stresses affecting your own life. The time analysis chart in Table 3-2 is a starting point for listing personal stress factors. The first step in organizing a time management system is setting priorities. What is more important to you? What is it that you want to do? After considering this and filling in the form, list how you feel about the findings. This analysis provides a master plan for instituting a new time priority

TABLE 3-2.
TIME ANALYSIS

Calculate the approximate amount of time spent per week on the categories listed. Recalculate the desired hours on the right-hand list.

| Time Spent in These Activities | Actual Hours/Week | Desired Hours/Week |
| --- | --- | --- |
| Work | | |
| Sleeping | | |
| Eating | | |
| Commuting | | |
| Parent–child interaction | | |
| Spouse interaction | | |
| Food preparation | | |
| Shopping | | |
| Housework | | |
| Volunteering | | |
| Recreation | | |
| Physical activity | | |
| Other | | |

program. Recognition is the beginning of the resolution. The rest of the solution is dedication to the commitment. If physical exercise is important, for instance, a schedule must be adhered to that allocates time for the activity. If a busy physician waits until she has time, the time will never come.

## RELAXATION TECHNIQUES

Relaxation is a natural method for coping with stress. Relaxation should allow you to rest your body and mind from stress. Most people consider relaxing to be an evening of television, but sometimes the stress of watching a football game, for example, can put emotions on a slow boil. What is relaxing for one person may not be relaxing for another. Relaxation can be found in a great variety of activities that allow the mind to slow down and release those things that cause stress. Spending time relaxing is an acquired skill. Learned relaxation techniques, including meditation, biofeedback, progressive relaxation, and exercise, are valuable, positive coping mechanisms.

### Meditation

Meditation is the state of prolonged focusing on a subject or object. If the focus is on an object, the eyes remain open, but otherwise are closed. Meditation is usually done in the sitting position in a quiet atmosphere and may use as a focus specific bodily functions such as heart rate or breathing (McLean 1982).

The first popular therapeutic relaxation was transcendental meditation (TM) (Walis 1983). Physiological studies have shown that TM can produce marked changes in the body, called the relaxation response, including a decrease in heart rate, a lowering of blood pressure, and a reduction in oxygen consumption. If done 10 to 20 minutes once or twice a day, it has been shown to produce a lasting reduction in stress-related symptoms.

### Biofeedback

Biofeedback is the simple process of monitoring one or more of the bodily functions with electrical devices that translate the activity into a receivable signal. The theory of biofeedback is that when people can observe this signal, they can learn to control the function being monitored. Biofeedback is a rapidly expanding field, and many mail-order catalogues today contain instruments for home use. The devices measure a variety of responses, including blood pressure, body temperature, muscle tension, and the galvanic skin response (McLean 1982).

### Progressive Relaxation

A process similar to biofeedback is called progressive relaxation. It is based on the assumption that stress and anxiety are directly related to muscle tension. If stress caused the tightness of muscles, the relaxation of these muscles should reduce stress (McLean 1982). Progressive relaxation is usually attempted in a reclining position in a quiet room. It can take many hours of learning the exercises to become adept at rapid and complete progressive relaxation.

## Exercise

Exercise is a stress reducer. Its importance in an overall stress reduction program cannot be overemphasized. Exercise is a means of relaxation but must be tailored to the individual's health status. Exercise can be viewed as a natural response to the fight-or-flight reaction. Stress primes the body for action, and exercise expends the built-up energy. An added benefit of exercising regularly is cardiovascular fitness, which contributes to overall well-being. Studies have shown regular exercise to be an adjunctive therapy in the treatment of depression and hypertension (McLean 1982).

## Imaging

Also known as visualization, imaging uses mental images as a means of relaxation. After meditation, it is probably one of the oldest forms of relaxation. In this exercise vivid images associated with rest and tranquility are used as positive feedback messages to the rest of the body. These images act as cues to relax tense muscles (Goliszek 1992).

## Support Groups

Support groups offer many benefits, particularly for women medical students (Davidson 1978; Konanc 1979; Wineberg 1972). Groups have been found to be of great benefit in increasing the capacity of sustained friendships (Davidson 1978). Formalized groups in medical school have become enduring relationships among women classmates and increased their understanding of women's professional difficulties (Konanc 1979). As a result of group experience, there is usually an increased feeling of closeness and solidarity in the working arena. This has been accompanied by decreased feelings of threat and competitiveness. Outside of the group experience, there is usually a decrease in the use of negative coping mechanisms and an increase in the use of positive coping mechanisms (Kahn and Schaeffer 1981). Groups have also been preferred to individual psychotherapy. Physicians feel a decreased sense of being alone in their suffering (Lamberg 1999).

## Social Support

As noted by Blake and Vandiver (1988), social supports have a positive, direct effect on health. "Four prospective population-based studies have found higher mortality during follow-up periods ranging from 30 months to 12 years in adults with weak as compared to strong supports. . . . Several studies have found increased rates of psychological impairment, particularly depression, in people with poor supports." Both intimate, confiding relationships and acquaintances are important, with the intimate ones more important to health status (Belle 1987). Although this does not prove that increasing social supports in times of stress will improve the individual's outcome, it would appear that increased contacts with friends, family, and others can ameliorate perceived stress and positively affect health.

Women participate in more and larger social support networks than men (Cleary 1987). They tend to have more confidants, whereas men have fewer confidants and more casual acquaintances (Belle 1987). Although these attachments are generally positive, women's larger networks may produce additional strains when individuals in the network turn to them for support and help (Belle 1987), as women are much more likely to accept a call to help others (Wethington et al 1987). For example, an ill relative requiring substantial help with daily activities can be a source of stress. The stress of the social networks, however, was found to be greater for women with fewer other resources, such as education and money (Belle 1987). In other words, a larger support network was only helpful to women with a fair amount of other resources, which would generally be true of women physicians. Thus, women's tendency toward intimate friendships and social contact may have a protective effect on health.

## Religion

Craigie et al (1988), in reviewing the literature, found that active involvement in a religion is associated with decreased morbidity and better physical and mental health. This effect may occur because of a variety of things, such as religious proscription of detrimental behaviors, increased levels of social support, and commitment to a major life goal. Regardless of the mechanism, religion can be an important tool for stress prevention and management for many people.

## Professional Counseling

Even with the aid of these intervention techniques, some people will find themselves without the personal resources to cope successfully with the stress of their professional and personal life. A physician who is unable to learn sufficient coping techniques should consider psychotherapy. Physicians often fear obtaining professional help, but they should not hesitate to do so in order to prevent impairment.

## Coaches

A popular form of seeking help in the business community has been the use of coaches. This has also spilled over into medicine. There are currently about 2,000 coaches in the United States, and the number is doubling every year. Coaches are not consultants or therapists per se. They typically charge about $150 an hour to provide a sounding board, a reality check, or a different perspective. One of the most often asked questions by physicians is, "How do I recapture the joy in my practice?" (Glabman 1998). See *www.coachfederation. org.*

## Shared-Schedule Residencies

In 1976, Section 709 of the Health Professions Assistance Act mandated shared-schedule positions in residency programs for family practice, general internal medicine, and general pediatrics in institutions receiving federal assistance (Shapiro and Driscoli 1979). This was rescinded under the Reagan budget cuts in the summer of 1983 (Shapiro et al 1980). There are, however, four general types of shared-schedule residencies (Shapiro and Driscoli 1978):

1. Integrated continuing model. In this model, two residents are paired in one training slot. This is a prototype that follows the original guidelines set by the government. Both residents will work between two-thirds and three-quarters time, and night and weekend call would be divided on an alternating schedule.
2. Alternating time blocks. One resident may be off for six months and on for six months. There may be various lengths of time involved.
3. Night float. In this system, one of the residents is on night duty while the other resident is on during the day.
4. Variable schedule. Combination of the above.

In 1980, less than one-third of institutions responding to a survey reported options for some type of reduced schedule training in at least one specialty (Shapiro 1980). The reduced schedule training by special arrangement was by far the most popular among the program directors. Some program directors permit reduced schedules by special arrangement without the need to have someone with whom to share the schedule (Brunton and Ostergaard 1982).

It must be noted there are problems with shared-schedule or reduced-time residencies:

1. Concern about continuity of patient services (Brunton and Ostergaard 1982; Shapiro and Driscoli 1978).
2. Concern about the quality of education for the residents in such a situation.
3. This type of residency can be a financial burden for the medical institution because of providing full benefits for residents theoretically working only half-time (Shapiro and Driscoli 1978).
4. There is resentment, envy, and often open hostility by the full-time staff (Heins et al 1977; Shapiro and Driscoli 1978).
5. Many participating residents are actually working three-quarters time but receiving half-time pay.
6. The schedule leads to a significant delay in completing training.

On the other hand, there may be some benefits to the directors of medical programs that offer shared-schedule residencies. For example, a more interesting type of person might be attracted to medicine. In one survey, the directors stated that they might indeed find more experienced, intelligent, and responsible staff through shared-schedule flexible programs. Staff morale, in general, might improve. The ultimate benefactor might be society when the young physicians are given the opportunity to satisfactorily develop their personal and professional lives.

## PRACTICE ALTERNATIVES

The practice environment is a very important part of the solution to role strain and stress for the woman physician. There is very little written in the literature on the various practice styles available; however, several less well known, but feasible, styles known to be in use will be discussed here. The commonly discussed practice types, which attract many men and women, include solo practice group or partnership practice, institutional practice, and academia. Here are some less frequently discussed types:

### Shared or Part-Time Positions

With a shared position, each physician shares a variable percentages of the patient load and time in the office. An example would be one physician scheduling patients in the morning, and the other physician scheduling in the afternoon. That way each works half-time with a practice equivalent to one solo practitioner. Physicians can also work part-time, with the same schedule each week or alternating time arrangements, such as alternating six months working and six months not working. The major disadvantage to part-time positions is that the overhead and benefits are often a greater proportion of the income, and full-time benefits may not always be available. Few malpractice insurance companies permit part-time physicians to pay reduced rate premiums.

### Home Office

The home office arrangement tends to be opted for only by the solo practitioner. A woman usually chooses it for the convenience of being near home. However, the privacy of the physician is distinctly decreased because of the presence of patients and office personnel in the home. There is also isolation from the rest of the medical community because of the location of the practice. However, it is a reasonable and viable alternative for many women, particularly psychiatrists. It is also more common than many realize. A report from the mid-1980s noted there were more than 100 home offices in Montgomery County, Maryland alone (Voelker 1989).

### Child in the Office

Women physicians who have the opportunity to do so may opt to take their young children with them to the office. The usual arrangement is to have one exam room or office designated as the child's playroom. Job descriptions for the office personnel would include child-care responsibilities, or a specific individual could be hired to work in the office for child care. This allows for mother–child interaction whenever there is a free moment and is convenient for breast-feeding. This works best in a solo office situation and when the child is very young, or older and able to care for themselves or even help in the office.

## Practice with Spouse

This option is not often chosen but allows for whatever time constraints the couple decides are necessary for each individual. The biggest problem with this arrangement is on-call coverage. Unless other physicians are actively taking call, there is no time for the couple to be away together.

In the authors' experiences, women frequently find practicing with other women more congenial than practicing with men. Women more frequently have similar practice styles and beliefs, such as how much time to spend with patients and how to charge. Other women may be more tolerant of the requirements of motherhood. More women than men may be interested in alternative practice arrangements.

## SUMMARY

Ideally, everyone should identify her/his own personal stresses and the importance of these stresses. After an evaluation, a person must desire to change his/her stress level and response in order to develop a realistic plan to follow. Specific stress-reducing activities and options that are outlined here must be incorporated into daily life in order to successfully manage stress.

## CHAPTER 4

# Enjoying a Marriage or Partnership

Deborah I. Allen and Marjorie A. Bowman

## PHYSICIAN MARRIAGES

Cross-sectional statistics indicate that 75% of female physicians are married, 11% were previously married, and 14% have not married (AMA 1991). Fewer are married than men physicians: 89% of men physicians are married, 7% were previously married, and 5% have not married. More women physicians get divorced: in one study, 37% compared to 28% (Rollman et al 1997). About 90% of the women physicians who marry have a professional spouse, and about half marry another physician (Sobecks 1999). This is quite a switch from the turn of twentieth century, when most women physicians were single and the expectation was that a professional woman would remain single.

There is some question as to whether the medical personality itself contributes to being a poor marriage partner (Fine 1981). The adjectives usually used to describe the medical personality are *bright* and *energetic,* coupled with *goal oriented, detached,* and *dedicated to work.* These attributes may result in lack of committed time to anything other than work. The spouses of physicians frequently believe they are "living alone but with somebody." Another phrase frequently used is that physicians are "married to their careers" (Gerber 1983).

Early in a physician's marriage, both spouses may view as temporary the difficulty of blending personal and professional lives. Indeed, many problems may lessen when physicians complete their training and have more control over their lives. However, some problems may be more fundamental to the individuals in the marriage and the physicians and her/his spouse may falsely believe that the marriage will improve later, perpetually accepting delayed gratification. During medical school and residency, studies and supervisors are easy targets as the cause of marital problems. But the training does end, and the realization that the spouse or marriage will not change comes slowly. The psychology of postponement can ultimately prove to be the psychology of avoidance. The avoidance grows directly out of the compulsive traits of many physicians and their potential preference (often subconscious) for work over family life (Gabbard and Menninger 1989).

Gabbard and Menninger (1988) found that both physicians (predominantly male) and spouses in troubled marriages ranked the same issues as sources of conflict in the marriage. Both ranked "lack of time for fun, family, and self" as the leading source of conflict. Physicians see "time away from home at work" as a much more important source of conflict than their spouses do. Spouses considered lack of intimacy as a much more serious problem than did the physicians. This is not surprising since 90% of the spouses in the survey were female and intimacy is a central concern to women.

Gabbard and Menninger feel that the lack of time serves as a convenient excuse for most couples. They feel that this complaint serves the function of attributing conflicts in the marriage to factors outside of the marriage. Actual conflicts arise around differences in three areas: the need for intimacy (spouse needs more than physician), perception of problems in the relationship, and communication styles (e.g., females prefer talking, males prefer sex) (Scheier 1988).

---

*93% of the spouses of women physicians are employed full-time.*

---

Though the characteristics of the female spouse of the male physician are changing, the largest profession recorded by this group is still "homemaker." In the study done by Nadelson et al (1979) at Harvard over a 10-year period (1967 to 1977), they found that over 90% of the male physicians had a spouse who stayed at home. In a study of over 3,000 family physicians done by Ogle et al (1986), 74% of the husbands of female family physicians had earned graduate degrees as compared to 30% of the wives of male physicians. For males in this study, two-thirds of the wives were not employed outside the home. Only 13% were employed full-time. In contrast, 98.9% of the husbands of the female family physicians were employed full time. Wives of male physicians were least likely to be working outside of the home if there were young children in the family. The wife's likelihood of outside work decreased with each additional child. These trends were not present in the marriages of female physicians. Husbands of the female physicians were highly likely to be employed regardless of the number of children.

More recent American Medical Association (AMA) data indicate that 93% of the spouses of women physicians are employed, compared to about 45% of the spouses of men physicians. Significantly, this rate of the wife's employment was similar for men physicians over and under the age of 40, suggesting an unchanging pattern.

## FEMALE PHYSICIAN MARRIAGES

Marriage can help or hinder careers independent of gender. However, marriage has been seen as a greater potential support to male physicians but more of a potential burden for female physicians (Vincent 1976). In one study, women physicians over age 45 scored their husbands as being somewhat unsupportive and against their careers (Parker and Jones 1981). Two to three times as many women physicians as men physicians expect to make career changes to accommodate a spouse's career (Kaplan 1970; Warde et al 1996). More men physicians report their spouse is extremely supportive of their career [79% compared to 69% of women physicians (Warde et al 1996) or 85% compared to 73% (Warde et al 1999)].

Conversely, some theorize that being married is a powerful, positive factor for men physicians and helps them buffer against many problems, including psychiatric disorders (Eisenberg 1981). In the general population, married men experience lower rates of depression and are healthier than single, separated, or divorced men (Cleary 1987; Eisenberg 1981). Alternatively, marriage does not have a protective effect on health for women (Cleary 1987), but employment does (Barnett et al 1987). Unfortunately, however, for mothers, the health advantage of being employed is negated if the husband does not participate in child care (Barnett et al 1987).

---

*Remember, even as a physician, "you will probably not prove to be [an] exception to any of the typical struggles that characterize marriage and family life" (Sotile and Sotile 2000).*

---

In a 1999 study of married physicians, Warde found that 63% of males were satisfied with their marriages as compared to 45% of the females. Higher satisfaction ratings were associated with a supportive spouse, little role conflict, salaried practices, and being married to a professional or a homemaker. In contrast, in a study in 1990 Spendlove et al did not find that women resident physicians experience more difficulties than men physicians in their marriages and found that resident physicians were as satisfied with their marriages as new attorneys.

The husband who is supportive of the woman pursuing a medical career will tend to be supportive of her in general and more responsible for domestic and parental responsibilities. If the female physician has a supportive husband, she will be more satisfied in her medical practice and less likely to work reduced hours (Parker and Jones 1981). In general, a supportive husband, rather

> Women physicians should not feel guilty about wanting equality on the home front. The most important single factor in the career of a married woman physician is the man she marries. Women physicians need to stand back and let their husbands take substantial responsibility for household management (Angell 1982). If a man begins to share household responsibilities and does a poor job, women may dive in and take over or criticize, discouraging further efforts. Men must be allowed to assume responsibilities in their own way. If a man does not cook or clean in the exact manner that the wife expects of him, perhaps the expectation should be changed (Angell 1982). Also, if such responsibilities are a new experience for him, he may improve with time as he learns how to better do the chores.

than just a husband, is important to the emotional health of the women (Belle 1987). The quality of the marriage is the key (Wethington et al 1987). Rather obviously, the choice of a husband may be one of the most significant choices any woman, including women physicians, can make. Women physicians desiring to marry deserve and need a supportive marital partner.

Myers (1984) claims that some women who study medicine have not grown up with a comfortable sense of themselves as being appealing or attractive to men. For these women, their scholastic achievement and ambition alone set them apart from peers of both sexes. The person who is unsure of themselves as humans will feel inferior in a marriage. They may be uncomfortable asserting themselves for fear of losing their spouse. Myers also believes that guilt is always present in women doctors with marital problems. He does not mean the normal guilt experienced by all perfectionistic women, but high levels of guilt that can lead to anxiety attacks and depressive symptomatology. The woman physician often feels that if she just worked a little harder, she alone should be able to correct the problems of the marriage.

One stress that may be especially problematic for women physicians is that they constantly give of themselves as a major nurturer both at home and at the office. When work is done, a married woman physician arrives home and may be expected by her family and herself to be a loving, supportive wife and mother. In contrast, a man often arrives home to his major source of emotional support (his wife) and may not be expected to be as giving emotionally. Clearly, these expectations may leave the woman with reduced energy for self-nurturance (McKay et al 1986).

## DUAL-CAREER MARRIAGES

Dual-career marriages are almost the norm in U.S. society and are certainly so for women physicians. Men need not be threatened by career wives and should be secure in their masculine identity. They must be able to assume responsibilities for household and child rearing as needed (Scott 1978). The personalities of those individuals who were found to have the highest role harmony in dual-career couples were those associated with higher levels of confidence in all areas, higher levels of adjustment, and relaxed, nonjudgmental perspectives (Cartwright 1978).

Social networks are important to the dual-career couple. Socializing for dual-career couples often involves other dual-career couples, appropriately so since this helps to reduce the pressure for "not being normal" and provides examples of how other couples manage. The couples may also have more in common. The wife's professional associates appear to be drawn into the social circles more of dual-career families than in a conventional middle-class family because of the need for societal support to sustain the dual-career pattern (Rapoport and Rapoport 1971).

Dual-career medical marriages can be wonderful. There are typically two people with reasonable to excellent social skills, intelligences, social commitment, incomes, persistence, and ability to commit. These qualities often make for an excellent marriage. However, there may be problems.

Some doctors tend to be authoritarian and find it hard to be democratic and egalitarian in a dual-career marriage (Fine 1981). One of the most important costs of a dual-career marriage is the time lost for spouse companionship. This cost may be borne equally by both partners. Some believe that women may feel the impact more since they may be socialized into roles that are more expressive and thereby may feel a greater need for dependency and affectionate feedback for maintenance of their self-esteem (Nadelson and Eisenberg 1977).

A second cost of the dual-career marriage may be the husband's ego identification. The male physician in a dual-career family may experience anxiety because he is not living up to his perceived expectation of the masculine role. He may be devalued by his friends, colleagues, or others, and perhaps by himself. The commonplace chores of domestic life can challenge even the liberated husband's commitment to an egalitarian marriage (Nadelson and Eisenberg 1977). However, many well-adjusted men experience considerable pride in their accomplished wives.

A third cost may be sexual problems. Johnson et al (1979) give case descriptions of sexual problems arising in dual-career families primarily related to shifts in the balance of power between the two spouses. The authors attribute some of the low sex drive of their dual-career patients to sheer exhaustion secondary to the much heavier than average work and family schedules. In several of the cases discussed, sexual dysfunction was used as a manipulative tool by the husband to express hostility toward the wife. Potter (1983) suggested that role strain in the marriage of two medical students leads to marital dysfunction with loss of sexual interest in the partner. The troubled physicians in Gabbard and Menninger's study (1988) conformed to the stereotype of being too busy and too tired to have sex. Frequency of sexual relations ranked high on the physician list as a source of conflict in the marriage. The mean frequency of sexual relations in this study was 1.6 times per week.

# DUAL-PHYSICIAN MARRIAGES

Dual-physician couples will become more of a phenomenon as more women continue to enter medical school. About half of married women physicians have a physician spouse (Sobecks et al 1999).

There are rewards to being married to another physician. After the training period, physician husbands and wives can be colleagues in practice and partners in continuing medical education (Lorber 1982; Sobecks et al 1999). The couples appear to become "helpmates" for each other in career matters. The physician spouse is often turned to for advice, and most dual-physician couples feel that the marriage is professionally beneficial. Both spouses appear to value a spouse who could understand their professional problems. Dual-physician couples also have higher incomes (Sobecks et al 1999).

There are also unique problems for the dual-physician marriages. The combined work hours are higher (Sobecks et al 1999). Women physicians married to men physicians work fewer average hours and average less income (Sobecks et al 1999) individually than other women physicians. They have more home responsibilities (Sobecks et al 1999, Tesch et al 1992). There are problems in trying to match internships, residencies, fellowships, and practices in the same location. After finding training sites, there is a tendency in dual-physician couples for one physician's career (often the man's) to dominate over the other (Tesch et al 1992). In virtually all cases studied prior to 1980 (Winter 1983), the husband's career determined where the family lived and worked. Johnson (et al 1979), found husband's careers typically took preference over the wife's career. As an example in the Johnson et al study, 67% of the men were in the specialty of their choice as compared to 45% of their spouses. Even in more recent studies, Tesch et al (1992) found that women married to physicians were twice as likely as women married to nonphysicians to interrupt their careers to accommodate their partner's careers: 27% of women physicians married to other physicians reported their spouse's career took preference; 35% of men physicians married to women admitted their own career took priority. Only 5% of women physicians married to other physicians felt their own career took priority (Sobecks et al 1999). Sobecks et al (1999) also found that women physicians married to other physicians were more likely to limit professional life for family reasons; one-third reported doing so, whereas only 15% of those women physicians with a spouse unemployed outside the home reported doing so. Only 7% of men reported limiting their professional life for family reasons.

Eisenberg (1981) claims that the lower academic ranking of women's professional careers stems from the geographic restriction imposed by a two-career household and the greater likelihood of women physicians being in a such a household. This is supported by the fact that married women physicians lag behind single woman physicians, as well as behind men, in academic advancements (Eisenberg 1981), although there may also be other mitigating factors (see Chapter 12).

In addition to the potential problems on the professional front, there are also those in the home environment. The question that may be most often asked in every dual-career family is who will handle the administrative functions of the family such as staying home to deal with repair people, serving as a chauffeur to the children, and being chief cook. Dual-physician families tend to have their children in a compressed period with little interrupted work by either spouse, accentuating the purely administrative hassles related to the family. Again, Tesch et al (1992) found that women physicians who were married to physicians, as compared to nonphysicians, spent more time with household responsibilities and worked fewer hours; in the WPHS, women physicians married to other physicians spent more time in child care and cooking (Frank et al 2000).

Gabbard and Menninger (1989) feel that the best way to support and save a physician-physician marriage is by preventive measures. Both physicians must realize that the marriage requires the attention of both partners. It can be the main source of coping with the stress of medical practice, as well as the first potential casualty of that stress. After identifying the need for attention to the marriage, each spouse needs to verbalize his or her needs and expectations from the union. Too many couples rely on mind reading. These authors recommend a mandatory time each day when spouses must sit down and discuss activities and plans. Attention must be paid to the quality of the conversation also. The needs of each partner must be made explicit.

---

*"In 'two-career' couples, the woman often has merely a job"*
*(Carol Kleeiman, Philadelphia Inquirer, Monday, March 13, 2000),*
*while the husband has a career. The women are more likely to*
*scale back their hours and move for their husband's job relocation.*

---

Heins (1982) suggests that husbands can help decrease some of the stress of the dual-doctor marriage by talking to their male colleagues about their home responsibilities. Children have been a forbidden topic of conversation at work for men, and there seems to be a sense of shame when it is necessary to leave work to do something for the family. It will be impossible for medicine to be sensitive to the needs of the family if physicians tend to deny and not discuss these needs (Heins 1982). If men physicians share their wife physician's concerns as spouses and parents, it might help legitimize certain issues that are currently shrugged off as merely women's issues (Angell 1982).

The final ingredient is the realization that no solution will be perfect. Most perfectionistic people (such as doctors) often assume that there is a perfect arrangement for every problem. A more realistic view would be that it is impossible to please everyone when trying to balance family and work life. The only solution is compromise. Each partner must make compromises in the direction of meeting the needs of the other person.

# THE NAME OF THE MARRIED WOMAN PHYSICIAN

When a woman marries, what should she do with her name? The male physician rarely has to concern himself with what he will be called when he is married, but marriage is a decision point for women. Not assuming her partner's name is often perceived as a lack of commitment to the marriage and to the spouse's family. Dralle (1987) found in her study that 18% of married female physicians did not change their names, and 64% took their husband's name. Another 16% used nontraditional variations of their names. She found that name changes had no connection to commitment to the marriage or satisfaction with their current name. She found that women who entered medicine when there were fewer women tended to keep their maiden names.

Thompson (1980) found the following problems tend to arise if a woman changes her name after she has established herself educationally, all of which remain true today:

1. If a woman changes her name with marriage, and has written and published articles, she could have two or more names referenced in Index Medicus.

2. Those who hyphenate their names find that the Library of Congress may classify a married woman under her husband's surname.

3. Some people will have trouble remembering the recently married woman's new name.

4. If a physician's diploma is issued in her birth name and she later marries, she may want to change her diploma, which is a major undertaking.

5. Patients may see diplomas and certificates in birth names and raise questions about their doctor's credentials.

6. If the physician divorces and remarries, the name problem becomes compounded.

# TIME AND DUAL CAREERS

Time is simultaneously the most precious commodity and the greatest source of stress to any physician. To successfully accommodate a dual-career family, the couple must judiciously allocate time. Time will become more precious than money for them, and spending money to relieve the couple of chores may provide more time for family life. Allocation of time can be done by establishing priorities and goals, both long-term and short-term. Time management is very important. Scheduling should be done on a weekly basis so that each knows the activities of the other, but monthly and yearly activities must also be planned. A large wall calendar with erasable surfaces is very helpful! It may be necessary for both of the partners to limit work in order to have the number of nonwork hours needed to meet the goals of the couple. Some couples spend one weekend a month away from home just to nurture their relationship (Scott 1978).

# THE IMPACT OF THE RISING NUMBER OF DUAL-PHYSICIAN COUPLES IN MEDICINE

With what is known about physicians, several outcomes could be expected from the rising number of dual-career couples in medicine. First, it could negatively affect the geographic distribution of physicians. It is generally easier for both individuals in a dual-career marriage to find satisfying work in large metropolitan areas. This could exaggerate the tendency of physicians to locate in urban rather than rural areas. Second, increasing numbers of dual-physician couples could decrease the number of physicians, particularly women, belonging to professional organizations. Women may be less likely to join organizations if their husbands belong. Third, overall productivity of physicians could decrease. As more physicians have higher-earning spouses, perhaps fewer will feel economic motivation to work longer hours. There may also be more interest in having sufficient home, leisure, and family time. Fourth, more systems to cater to dual-career couples will be developed. This may mean more family-options benefit packages and support systems at organizations that hire physicians.

**On Being Single.**
Singlehood can provide more freedom and permit more self-sufficiency, and can be quite rewarding (Notman 1988 and Nadelson).

Women physicians may make a conscious decision to be single, by never marrying or seeking divorce. Being single does not necessarily mean the lack of a partner, as many single women have partners. With or without partners, many of the stresses and joys of being a woman physician are similar.

Single women physicians have often reported to us that the most common problems they have based on their singlehood are the presumptions other people make about them. A very common presumption is that single women physicians have no commitments outside of work; i.e., they must always be free to fill in for someone else at the last minute, or certainly they can stay late, or it is okay to give them a disproportionate share of the work load. Single women physicians report they have many commitments outside of work, often with family, church, or other activities, or to themselves and the time they need alone. Another presumption relates to the expectation that they have a spouse or partner, or that social activities are geared to physicians *and* their spouses.

Single women can make the female spouses of men physicians uncomfortable. It may be harder for a nonworking spouse to relate to a women who does not have a husband and children to care for, and there is always the potential of the development of male–female relationships (however, this is not limited to single individuals!). A lesbian partnership, certainly more accepted than in the past, is also not the norm and may create anxiety in others.

*(continued)*

*(continued)*

Just as we should not stereotype physicians of minority races, married physicians, female physicians, or other subsets, we should not stereotype single physicians.

## SUMMARY

Marriage and partnerships have many internal benefits for women physicians but also create new and different stresses. The choice of a husband/partner is paramount, and the more supportive the partner, the better the mental health of the women physician. Marrying a husband with his own career likewise adds additional constraints, particularly on the geographic moves sometimes needed for career advancement, time for leisure activities, and the complexity of household management. However, marrying another professional or physician increases income and may provide additional support in learning from each other's experience. While considering all of the factors, specific attention must be paid to the relationship of the partners to each other to allow maximal personal fulfillment for both.

## CHAPTER 5

# The Second Shift

Meredith Mitchell, Marjorie A. Bowman,
and Erica Frank

Female and male physicians share many joys and stresses, but women physicians may be more involved with the tasks of domestic life.

In studies of physician stress, men are more likely to cite issues related to work and women to cite their home life. For example, in a study of 33 male and 39 female physicians of various specialties, male physicians said their stressors were mostly from professional concerns such as malpractice, inability to cure, and doctor–patient relationships. The women physicians in the study were much more likely than the men physicians to feel stressed about career/family conflict (44% vs. 6%) (Gross 1992). A survey of 667 women and men physicians also found that women perceived lack of time for family as a problem, whereas men physicians were more concerned with patient interactions, malpractice, and peer review (Hojat et al 1995). In yet another study, between 58% and 78% of women physicians experienced conflict between work and home life (Tesch et al 1992). Women and men physicians seem to experience similar stresses associated with their medical training and careers; however, women physicians may also feel pressure to mesh their careers with the stresses of traditional women's roles.

One solution could be to avoid some of the issues by not marrying or having children. Although single women often still have family and other outside obligations, women physicians who are single and childless (or with fewer children) unsurprisingly spend less time on housework and cooking (Frank and Harvey 2000). However, most women physicians have a career and a family life. According to 1989 AMA data, 14% of women physicians compared to 5% of men physicians have never married, and 93% of men physicians have had children compared to 85% of women physicians (AMA 1991). (These data are not adjusted for women physicians being younger, on average, than male physicians.)

## DOMESTIC RESPONSIBILITIES

Housework and child care—somebody has to do them. Though women have come a long way in many avenues of medicine, they still have a long way to go at home. The Women Physicians' Health Study (WPHS) found that the average woman physician spent 24.4 hours a week on child care, a half hour a day on cooking and a half hour a day on housework. [Most of the data in this chapter derived from WPHS can be found in more detail in Frank and Harvey (2000).] Not surprisingly those with more domestic responsibilities were likely to work fewer clinical hours. The women physicians who cooked more and did more housework reported higher levels of stress at home, but lighter work stress. Overall, women physicians spend little time as compared to other women on domestic activities that can be done by others, such as cooking and housework.

---

*Between work and home, women physicians worked 22 hours more per week than men physicians.*

---

Woodward et al (1996) found in a study of over 400 physicians that women physicians worked 40 hours a week on child care. Men physicians worked slightly over 11 hours a week on child care. Including hours spent at work, women physicians worked 22 hours more a week than men physicians. In this study 30% of the women worked full time and 85% of the men worked full time.

---

*Average fathers in intact families do not do as much child care as average mothers. On weekdays, typical fathers give sons more attention than daughters. The higher the mother's income, the more time the father usually contributes to child care on the weekend. (Elias M. Fathers focus increased care on boys.* USA Today *June 14, 1999, page D6.)*

---

Both the numbers of hours of total housework per week and the percentage of housework is important to women's mental health (Bird 1999; Schwartzberg and Dytell 1996). In a large study of nonphysicians, Bird (1999) found that increasing numbers of hours spent in housework were

*(continued)*

*(continued)*
associated with small increases in depression and mental distress. However, even more important was the percentage of housework. For working women, those who reported the housework activity to be fairly evenly divided had the least distress. Unfortunately, the average women who did not report keeping house full-time (meaning women who were in school, retired, or employed full-time or part-time) reported performing about 65% of the work. Men reported about 43% of the work. Thus men were closer to that magical 50-50 than were women. (It is also quite noticeable that the totals between the men and women are greater than 100%. The author notes other studies that indicate that men underestimate the amount of work done by others.) The women had significantly higher levels of depression and distress that was almost entirely accounted for by inequity in household labor division.

In 1992, Brown found that 65% of the 62 Canadian women family physicians she studied were overwhelmed at least once a week by their multiple responsibilities. Unlike previous studies, she found that despite their feelings of being overwhelmed, they all functioned well and maintained high levels of self-esteem. Those who were seldom overwhelmed spent an average of 37 hours a week working. Women who were overwhelmed spent an average of 43 hours a week at work. It is possible that these 6 hours make a substantial difference: those critical 6 hours may be a strategic boundary between being overwhelmed and being in control. All the women in this study felt that they did not have enough time to spend on friends. However, larger studies have shown that women physicians work an average of 52 hours per week (AMA 1998), putting most of them, according to these results, at risk for burnout.

Women physicians expect equal sharing of child care and household responsibilities, whereas men expect to contribute less than their wives do to these tasks (Kaplan 1970). Nonphysician fathers who do care more for children in the mother's absence rate their marriages more poorly (Barnett et al 1987) than do others, and this may well be true for physician fathers. Despite high expectations, women continue to bear the major responsibilities for the family and home. If male partners are helpful in the home, they are often self-congratulatory and awarded accolades for the effort (Nadelson and Eisenberg 1977) but may suffer more depression (Barnett et al 1987).

We hope that the inequality is changing. There seems to be some indication that men are diminishing their intense career commitment and increasing their level of family involvement, whereas women appear to be going in the opposite direction (Eisenberg 1981). In a 1988 study, women physicians with physician-partners still in training had a more equal household task distribution than those women physicians with physician-partners already in practice (Tesch et al 1992). This could indicate that younger couples have a more egalitarian attitude toward domestic activities; however it could also be an effect of having dif-

The simplistic answer list:
1. Hire help.
2. Hire more help.
3. Hire even more help.
4. Talk.
5. Talk some more.
6. Talk in a better way.
7. Forget all that, and forget all the housework.

ferent schedules because of training or having fewer or no children. This is also suggested by some convergence in female and male physician's productivity.

In an older study, 30% of women physicians had no domestic help (Heins et al 1977). Seventy-six percent of the respondents did all the cooking, shopping, child care, and money management for the household. Even in dual-career marriages, women continued to be responsible for the children, regardless of their level of professional commitment (Eisenberg 1981). The responsibility for household work is compounded by the difficulty in finding qualified household help or by the available help being unskilled in child care. Frequently the available child care is from a different economic or educational class or a different background and has different child-rearing practices than the physician (Heins 1982).

Another aspect of stress related to home or work life is time-sensitive work. In the home where domestic work is divided, it remains common for the woman to have the time-sensitive chores—those chores that must be done in a relatively short, specific time frame, such as getting the kids ready for school or picked up from day care by a set hour, or getting dinner ready, whereas men have traditionally had chores for which the time of accomplishment is less specific, such as mowing the lawn, or doing the family finances. A study by Sullivan (1997) used time diaries to quantify the amount of time men and women spend on domestic activities. He found that the tasks men spent the most time on were gardening and odd jobs or do-it-yourself work, chores that can be saved for the weekend or other free time, whereas women's top three tasks were cooking, cleaning, and clothes care. He also found that men are more likely to perform household tasks with their partner, whereas women are more likely to do them alone.

## Cooking

Women physicians average less than 30 minutes of cooking time per day (Frank and Harvey 2000). This is significantly less than most women, even those who work full-time. Homemakers spend an average of about 12.1 hours per week on cooking, women who work part-time average 10.9 hours cooking per week, and women who work full-time average 8.6 hours per week (Shelton 1992). The average for women physicians is only about 3.1 hours per week. Cooking seems to be especially expendable to women physicians!

---

*Women physicians spend 3 hours per week cooking versus*
*9 hours spent by other women who work full time.*

---

Women physicians choose to delegate goods (prepared foods) or a service (food preparation) because it is a low priority. Physicians probably spend less time cooking because they can afford other options such as eating out, ready-made meals, or hiring help.

Physicians who cooked more tended to be married to a more educated husband (including husbands who are also physicians), have more children, take fewer nights of call, be less likely to work professionally, and have more home stress and less work stress (Frank and Harvey 2000). Meal preparation is a time-sensitive domestic activity. Meals take place at approximately the same time and on a daily basis. These time constraints cause more stress at home. However, if a physician had more time for planned, daily activities like meal preparation, then she would be more likely to have a less stressful, more regular professional life. Among the specialties, surgical subspecialists cooked the least, whereas anesthesiologists, emergency medicine physicians, and general practitioners cooked the most (Frank and Harvey 2000).

Nondrinkers and women who exercised more spent more time cooking, possibly because they are more health conscious or have generally allocated more time for self-improvement and nonwork activities (Frank and Harvey 2000). Not surprisingly, physicians who cooked less were more likely to be in a solo or two-person practice, to work more hours, and to earn more money, or were the only wage earner in the household (Frank and Harvey 2000).

## Housework

Women physicians spend about the same amount of time on housework as they do on cooking—less than 30 minutes per day, for a total of 2.9 hours per week. This represents an even more pronounced difference than the practice of other women. In one study, homemakers spent 24.3 hours per week, women employed part-time spent 20.7 hours per week, and women employed full-time spent 18.3 hours on housework (Shelton 1992). This is most likely because housework is even easier to commission than is cooking and may be a less enjoyable activity. Similar to the profile of those who cooked, physicians with more educated husbands, fewer nights on call, or lower personal income spent more time doing housework. Again, more time spent on housework was correlated with more stress at home. As with cooking, surgical subspecialists spent the least time per week (1.2 hours) and general practitioners spent the most (5.0 hours) on housework.

## Child Care

One aspect of domestic activity where women physicians are more comparable with the general population is child care. Women physicians tend to spend about 24 hours a week in child care (Frank and Harvey 2000). This is slightly less than the average for employed U.S. mothers in dual-parent households. Nock and Kingston gathered complete data on the subject by using diaries of seven different child care activities and found that working mothers usually spent 4 hours each workday and 8 hours on Sunday with children younger than school age, and 4 hours each workday and 6 hours on Sunday with children older than preschool. Women physicians average just under 4 hours per day in child care. Therefore, women physicians spend somewhat less time with their children as compared to other working women, likely due to a combination of higher career satisfaction, greater relative financial rewards for working, busier and more erratic schedules, and the ability to pay for higher quality child care. However, child rearing differences between women physicians and other working women is much smaller than for other domestic responsibilities, suggesting that women physicians consider child rearing to be a more important, more enjoyable, and/or less transferable task.

Among women physicians, those that were married to a physician, whose spouse made more money, and who had lower personal income tended to spend more time on child care (Frank and Harvey 2000). Many of these are predictable findings. If one spouse is bringing in more money, then there is less pressure for the other to work as much, and more time is available for high priority domestic responsibilities such as child care.

Physicians who were younger, worked less than 40 hours per week, and were professionally inactive also spent more time on child care (Frank and Harvey 2000). Again, this makes sense: younger women likely have younger children who need more care, and women working part-time or not at all may have done so in order to spend more time with their children. However, only 2% of the 1,297 women physicians in WPHS with children under 18 were professionally inactive (Frank and Harvey 2000). A Canadian study showed that 55% of women physicians versus 19% of men physicians had taken a break from education or practice since graduation from medical school; there was an 18-fold difference between women and men in whether or not these breaks were related to children (Bryant et al 1991). Several studies have shown that women with children are more likely to work fewer hours (Bryant et al 1991; Frank and Harvey 2000; Tesch et al 1992; Uhlenberg and Cooney 1990). A Canadian study found that nearly half of the women physicians with children saw patients <30 hours per week, whereas only 17% percent of both men and women physicians without children saw patients <30 hours per week (Bryant et al 1991).

Characteristics that did not correlate with the amount of time spent on child care were exercise habits, marital status, sexual identity, home or work stress, specialty, career satisfaction, practice locale, number of nights on call, or days lost to bad physical or mental health (Frank and Harvey 2000). Some of these characteristics seem to be unrelated to time spent with children, but others seem to have an impact on it. For example, a physician with many on-call nights may have less predictable free time to spend with children. Also, one's specialty could affect the amount of time with children, because some specialties require erratic hours or emergencies, whereas others are more routinely scheduled and allow room for planning. All of this suggests the high importance women physicians place on spending time with their children.

## LEISURE TIME

Gardening is not a high-priority activity for women physicians; they averaged only 3 minutes a week on gardening. Even though older, widowed, and rural physicians tend to garden more, they still only average 20 minutes to a half hour per week. This is probably because it is an activity that is easily avoided or hired out.

Gardening also may be considered leisure, which in the busy schedule of a woman physician with a family is one of the first things given up. Lorber (1982) found this in interviews with women physicians; they were more likely to give up free time than work in order to spend time with children. It has also been shown that women have less leisure time than men in the general population (Shelton 1992). Whereas men spend more time on paid work and leisure, women spend more time on domestic or combined domestic activities (Sullivan 1997). In addition, women are more likely than men to combine tasks, for instance, washing dishes while clothes are drying and keeping an ear out for the children, which makes women's household labor more intense (Sullivan 1997).

Another stress can be that not only do women have less leisure time than men, it often is not of as good quality. Women's leisure is much more likely to be interrupted and is more likely to be interrupted by domestic work (Sullivan 1997). Therefore, although reading a book can be considered a leisure activity, frequently the reading may occur while clothes are washing or children are napping or playing, and will be interrupted easily and frequently. This may be because mothers allow themselves to be interrupted more than fathers.

## ROLE STRAIN

Role strain for the woman physician is the conflict that results from having to choose between the multiple demands placed on her by her profession and those that arise from her obligations as a mother, a wife, and a person in her own right (Pfeiffer 1983).

The Women Physicians' Health Study is the largest examination of this phenomenon. Contrary to conventional wisdom, WPHS found that those women physicians with children were more likely to be satisfied with their career choice than were those without children. Further, WPHS found a positive linear and significant ($p < .0001$) association between the number of children and career satisfaction. Among postmenopausal women (e.g., those who had achieved their ultimate family sizes), 90% of physicians with four or more children were satisfied with their career versus 73% of those without children.

Others have found less encouraging results. In a study of over 1,400 physicians, Warde et al (1996) looked at role conflict by age and gender. They found that 87% of female physicians and 62% of male physicians experienced role conflict. Unlike previous studies, they also found that many men do experience "moderate" role strain. In the same study, 85% of the women made career changes for their children, most notably decreasing their work hours. Only 28% of the men made similar changes. According to Aneshensel and Pearlin (1987), inter-role conflict is greater when family role demands are extreme or inflexible, or commitment to work is strong.

Similarly, in comparison to men physicians, women physicians experience more role strain in the areas of child care, household responsibilities, and marriage commitments (Cohen et al 1988). In one study (Cartwright 1978), 51% of female physicians felt some intermittent role strain and 20% experienced much strain. Only a third had achieved what they felt to be harmonious integration of their roles. The two variables that related negatively to role harmony were the number of children and the women's age; i.e., the more children or the older the woman physician, the greater the role strain.

In their book *Gender and Stress*, Barnett et al (1987) conclude that women are inherently more stressed than men, due primarily to the role of mother, which has high demands and is low on control. In contrast, the role of father is traditionally low in demands and high in control. They go on to say, "Indeed, the price of being a fully socialized female in our culture may be a predisposition to feelings of lack of control and ultimately to depression" (p. 358). According to these authors, the negative effect of being a mother, particularly a mother of preschool or numerous children, had more of an effect on well-being than did working or marriage.

Most women physicians combine family, career, and the experience of pregnancy at some time during their medical careers (Bonar et al 1982). The juggling act that this requires is often most intense in the woman's thirties. This is a time when career development is most rapid for men, but women physicians are likely to be in the midst of raising her young children as well as developing her career (Angell 1982). It is difficult for the woman physician not to compare herself and her career development with that of men.

## THE BOTTOM LINE

Patterns show that the more a women physician earns or works at her job compared to her husband, the less responsibility she has at home for cooking, cleaning, and child care. Nearly all women physicians (93%) are married to someone who works outside of the house (AMA 1991). The census data also shows that women physicians married men physicians in the same numbers in

---

### Vignette: Life Balancing:
### Combining a Career and Personal Life in a Mutually Enriching Way

I married at the age of 20 after my first year of medical school and had four children over the next decade while completing medical school, a psychiatry residency, and child psychiatry fellowship, and beginning a career in academic psychiatry. As one might imagine, I had considerable interest in finding models of ways to successfully combine career and a family and personal life. For 10 years (from 1981 to 1991) I co-taught a lunchtime elective for first-year medical students called "Parenting and Professionalism: Combining Career and Family." We learned from each other, from the literature, and from guest panelists of physicians with different specialties, as well as from spouses and children of physicians. We distilled the following basic principles:

1. Define your personal and professional life priorities in conjunction with your significant others. Be flexible about changing priorities over the life cycle as circumstances change.

2. Sustain and nurture relationships with significant others. "Quality time" by necessity involves quantity of time.

3. Organize, plan, schedule, share responsibilities, and delegate to others both at work and at home. You don't have to do everything yourself.

4. Find outlets for stress reduction: exercise, relaxation, hobbies, and socializing, and maintain a sense of humor.

5. There are still gender differences. Women continue to more commonly assume major family executive responsibilities and to experience more role strain and conflict than men, whether for biologic, societal, or psychosocial reasons, or all three. Men who wish to have more involvement with families or other personal interests are often under pressure to perform in their careers and may lack role models and support for better life balancing.

6. Be aware how the traditional lifestyle and personality styles of physicians (combinations of conscientiousness, perfectionism, and nurturing behaviors) affect efforts at life balancing, on relationships, and on the choice we make.

*Diane K. Shrier*

---

1980 as they did in 1995 (50%). In these dual-physician marriages, 73% of the time the physician husband earns more money and 63% of the time he works more hours than does the physician wife (Uhlenberg and Cooney 1990).

---

*Women physicians spend more time on housework if married
to another physician rather than to a nonphysician.*

A 1988 study of 247 women physicians showed that women physicians married to a physician were more likely to take primary responsibility for more household tasks, than were women physicians married to nonphysicians (Tesch et al 1992). The study also found that women physicians partnered to nonphysicians worked more outside the home and their spouses worked less compared to dual-physician marriages, in which the physician husband usually works more than the physician wife (Tesch et al 1992). A British study found that 50% more women physicians that men physicians felt that children had interrupted their careers, and although only 2% of men physicians reported doing the primary shopping or cooking, 80% of women physicians reported taking sole responsibility for these tasks in their households (Uhlenberg and Cooney 1990).

Women physicians tend to neglect or delegate other things in order to spend time on work and with children, or make adjustments in their type of work to accommodate children. Not many women physicians with children are professionally inactive, but they often work fewer hours. Also, although they may spend slightly less time with their children than the average American mother, they spend substantially less time on all other household activities.

---

*Time spent on domestic activities is not related to
career satisfaction or health.*

---

Possibly the most important thing to mention about the domestic activities of women physicians is that in the WPHS survey of 4,500 women physicians, the amount of time spent on domestic activities was not correlated with career satisfaction or with physical and mental health (Frank and Harvey 2000). Women physicians' paths to happiness do not seem to rely on 'doing it all'; delegation works.

## CHAPTER 6

# HAVING AND RAISING CHILDREN

MARJORIE A. BOWMAN AND DEBORAH I. ALLEN

It is generally accepted and expected that most people and most physicians (men and women) will have children. There is some converse acceptance for women, particularly professional women, to have no children. A woman physician makes a decision whether to have children. Does she want them? If so, when? What will be the sacrifices, the problems? How will she and her family manage?

In the 1994 Women Physicians' Health Study (WPHS) survey, about 70% of all women physicians ages 30 to 70 report having children and the mean number of children was 1.6 (Frank et al 1997). Surgeons were less likely to have children or had fewer children. Women physicians are less likely to have children than are men physicians. Warde et al (1999) found 73% of responding women physicians and 90% of men physicians in Southern California in 1988 had children. In a 1995 nationwide survey, 69% of academic women and 84% of academic men physicians had children; the women also averaged fewer children—2.1 compared to 2.5 children (Carr et al 1998). The American Medical Association (1991) found that 92% of women physicians and 96% of men physicians over the age of 50 had had at least one child.

## BEING A PHYSICIAN AND MOTHER

In some ways, there appears to be much in common between being a physician and being a mother. A physician is caring, dedicated, and works long hours. The same is true of a mother. Both must set priorities. Both listen and help others to understand, to figure things out, and move ahead with their lives. Both are important to society. Both are healers. Both feel guilty if they do not devote enough time or effort to their perceived duties.

Conversely, the two roles are also different. One provides financial rewards; the other takes them away. One enables you to buy material goods; the other destroys them, such as when a child throws a ball and breaks the mother's favorite piece of pottery. One exalts you in public; the other role is generally a private activity that sometimes brings public embarrassment, such as the naively rude public statement or temper tantrum by a toddler. Both are careers, however, and not simply jobs.

In WPHS, women physicians who themselves spent fewer hours performing child care had more career satisfaction and more desire to be a doctor but less desire to remain in their specialty. Among those who had attained their ultimate family size (postmenopausal women, $n - 1,830$), there was a significant and linear association between the number of children and career satisfaction, with 90% of these physicians with four or more children satisfied with their career choice versus 73% of those with no children (Frank et al 1999). Maybe "having it all" *is* the answer!

## THE DECISION

The decision to have children is a very personal one. Clearly, the time and financial commitment inherent in child rearing means forced prioritization once children are born. It becomes more difficult to work a physician's 60 to 70 hours a week and still have time for oneself. One also never knows how one will personally react to the change in responsibilities—how much guilt will there be in combining career and parenthood? Children are ephemeral ideas—that is, until they are born. How one will handle the responsibilities, whether one will enjoy or hate the experience, is unknown until the child is physically present. Even then, one never knows what the next stage of the child's life will bring. Thus there will always be a certain amount of uncertainty; it is unavoidable.

## UNCERTAINTY

Becoming pregnant involves physical and emotional risk. The fact that many people have had children and thoroughly enjoyed the experience may be reassuring, but it does not guarantee that any one individual will react similarly, particularly a person who is different. The women physician has spent much of her life attaining her career goal. Having a family may always have seemed like a good idea, but what does it truly mean? Children can be the most fulfilling part of life, bringing great joy and satisfaction; they also can be very trying and emotionally distressing, both as young children and when older. Women ask themselves, will I have enough time, energy, and love to provide what I believe to be a good upbringing? Yes, I always thought I could do anything (I proved that by becoming a physician), but can I accept a role that is fulfilling internally (for its own sake), as compared to externally (for the good of mankind)? Will I enjoy a role whose rewards are more from direct interaction (children) than from the admiration of society and others ("She's so great—she's a physician!")?

## THE TIMING OF CHILDBEARING

The choice of when to have a baby is a very individual matter, although unplanned pregnancies also occur. Each career period during which a woman may have children is fraught with a variety of problems; each also has its unique benefits. The timing of childbearing is a personal decision each woman will have to make based on her own situation. However, even not deciding is a decision, because time marches on.

In WPHS (Frank and Cone 2000), there were 87 pregnant physicians. The average age was 34.1 years. Almost all (97%) were married. Their self-reported health status was better than that of the nonpregnant women physicians of the same age. Their number of work hours per week, career satisfaction, and work stress were similar to those of the same-age nonpregnant physicians.

## FACTORS IN TIMING CHILDREN

There are physiologic, career, and financial and personal factors in timing children.

### Physiologic

Women lose fertility as they age, with greater decrements in fertility at about age 35 years, and dramatic decreases after age 40 years, with the average menopause occurring at age 52 years in the United States.

Unplanned pregnancies are common even among knowledgeable women, partly as a result of imperfect birth control. Several studies have identified the frequency of unplanned pregnancies among women physicians. In Sinal et al's (1988) survey of 900 women physicians, 77% reported that their first pregnancies were planned.

## Pregnancy Complications and Outcomes

In a large study of pregnancy complications and outcomes in women physicians, Phelan (1988) analyzed the responses from 1,197 women physicians. She found that the actual rate of medical and obstetrical complications was no different from that in the general population, except that the incidence of pregnancy-induced hypertension was higher than in the general population (12% compared to 5%). The figures were not controlled for age, which could account for differences in hypertension rates. Osborn et al (1990) surveyed 92 residents and 144 spouses of residents nationally for pregnancy outcome. They identified an increased risk of premature labor among the Caucasian resident pregnancies. No significant differences were found in the rates of prematurity, spontaneous and therapeutic abortions, or congenital anomalies between the two groups, and the outcomes were similar to previously published figures for nonphysician pregnancies. In a national sample comparing the pregnancies of wives of male medical residents (1,238 in number) to those of women residents (989 in number), there was no difference in the rates of miscarriages, ectopic gestations, stillbirths, preterm births, or low birth weight babies (Klebanoff et al 1990). As in the Osborn study, women residents had more preterm labor, but not more preterm delivery. The study also found a higher rate of preeclampsia among the women residents and that women working more than 100 hours per week had a greater risk of preterm birth. In a study of 454 pregnancies of obstetricians (Greenbaum et al 1987), women having their first pregnancy during residency training had a statistically significant higher percentage of low birth weight infants than those having them later. Intrauterine growth retardation was also common (7.5%).

---

*In one study, women physicians working more than 100 hours per week had a greater risk of preterm birth.*

---

## Career

The timing options for women physicians' pregnancies are before medical school, during medical school, during residency, and while in practice. When asked retrospectively, most women physicians would recommend to others that they have children after completion of the residency (Sinal et al 1988).

> ## Vignette
>
> It's the things that you have always known that you take for granted. My mother was always a doctor, so as I was growing up I didn't think a lot about what it meant to have a physician mother. She just was. It was only when I reached medical school that I realized how fortunate I was. While my female peers were struggling with the issue of how to balance career and family, I was thinking, "I have it easy." First of all, I had peers. My mother had to overcome a predetermined quota for women to get into her medical school, while 40% of my class were women. She had four children during her medical education and early career, while the only diapers I saw were during my pediatric training. Mom broke the glass ceiling time and again, so I did not have to run up against it. It never occurred to me that I couldn't advance professionally and take on leadership positions in my field.
>
> Mom never pushed me to become a physician, but I know how proud she is that I chose to go into medicine. And I know how lucky I am to have a mother who also has been a remarkable role model.
>
> *Lydia A. Shrier*
>
> See page 42 for her mother's vignette

## Childbearing Before Medical School

### Pros

Psychologists Panmore, Daniet, and Winegarten of the Westlake College Center for Research on Women studied 86 couples and concluded the following were advantages of having children when a woman was in her twenties (Stephen 1983):

1. *More energy.* Women in their twenties have more energy and enthusiasm to spend on child rearing.
2. *Fewer nonchild responsibilities.* If the woman is not attending school during this time, there may be relatively few other infringements on her time, allowing more time for child rearing.
3. *Greater flexibility.* A woman in her early twenties is not as set in her ways as older women. This flexibility allows her to adjust to child rearing more readily.
4. *Less infringement on professional growth.* Having children before medical school means that pregnancy and childbirth will not interfere with medical school or professional career. (But child rearing might!)
5. *Less financial and professional impact of time out.* After a woman starts to earn money, the family tends to become more dependent on the steady source of income. If the woman has not as yet begun to earn a good income, then the financial impact may be less. Taking time out before one

is established in a career may also mean less loss of professional stature later.

6. *Physiologic maximization.* The twenties are the best physiologic time for having children.

7. *Greater maturity in medical school.* Entering medical school later than the average student provides for greater maturity and a greater understanding of the important aspects of the educational process.

*Cons*

1. *Greater isolation in medical school.* The older medical school student who is a parent may have less peer support and be more isolated (Bluestone 1965).

2. *Greater responsibilities.* Child care presents an additional responsibility and financial strain to those inherent in attending medical school.

3. *Lack of role models.* There are fewer role models for the woman medical student with children.

4. *Resentment by children.* Children may resent the mother's new time commitments and interests. This will vary from child to child, but a general rule would be that any major interest of this magnitude will draw resentment from children.

5. *Forced redirection upon entry to medical school.* The shift from child rearing to full-time study in medical school can be challenging. There will have to be a reorganization of priorities from child care to schoolwork in order to maintain good academic standing. The previous independence that had often been enjoyed by the student may create trouble in coping with the rigid and inflexible experience of medical training.

## Childbearing During Medical School

*Pros*
Many of the advantages of having a child before medical school, as discussed above, apply during medical school: more energy, greater flexibility, physiologic maximization (depending on age), and less financial and professional impact of time out.

*Cons*

1. *Losing academic time.* Medical schools can be rigid, though there are exceptions, and pregnancy with delivery during a school year may result in falling behind academically. Some medical students take no time off, whereas others had to repeat an entire academic year (Kaplan 1970).

2. *Lack of role models.* Not many others choose this route, making it difficult for individuals to observe and follow patterns set by role models.

3. *Discouragement.* There is often little encouragement, and often active discouragement, of medical students wishing to have children (Pfeiffer 1983).

4. *Multiple responsibilities.* This is self-evident.

5. *Forced redirection.* The forced redirection is from full-time student to full-time student and mother.

6. *Inhibition of identity development.* During her early training, the woman student is continuing to develop her own female identity while simultaneously trying to develop the identity of a physician (Ordway 1980). The establishment of the ego and sexual identities in a woman at this age may be postponed if she is overwhelmed by the combined tasks of motherhood and completing medical school (Pfeiffer 1983). The changes that occur during medical school may result in the desire for different roles than those originally expected when the student was younger.

7. *Financial burdens.* Unless there is a spouse with a high income or parents willing to support the efforts of the new family, the cost of medical school and child care during medical school may be prohibitive (Bluestone 1965).

8. *Peer resentment.* Peers may resent the student-mother's outside responsibilities or her need to change schedules (Potter 1983).

## Childbearing During Residency

### Pros

1. *Possibility of more flexible schedules.* There are flexible-schedule residencies available, although not many, and they frequently require the resident to help make the arrangements.

2. *Identity development more complete.* Much development of identity as a woman and as a physician will have occurred prior to residency (Ordway 1980; Pfeiffer 1983), and the woman will have made specific commitments to the profession.

3. *Physiologic maximixation.* If the woman is still in her twenties, physiology is on her side (Bluestone 1965).

4. *Reasonable energy levels.* Although a resident's energy level may be less than in her twenties, it will still be higher than in later years (Baucom-Copeland et al 1983; Bluestone 1965). However, residency time commitments can interfere considerably with this energy.

### Cons

1. *Prolongation of residency and resulting delay in board certification.* Maternity leaves, as well as other leaves for children's need and/or for disabilities, can result in a delay in residency graduation and in board certification for many specialties (Potter 1983). This delay is now more significant since many health maintenance organizations require board certification for their physicians.

2. *Peer resentment.* There is often resentment expressed by other residents if a pregnant resident or resident mother is given special considerations. In many instances, the pregnant resident has to make up on-call obligations by having a heavier call schedule before and/or after delivery; adjustment may be needed to allow the resident to be on more difficult rotations early in the pregnancy and less difficult rotations late in the pregnancy. This may create practical and emotional difficulties and conflicts with peers (Baucum-Copeland et al 1983; Klebanoff et al 1990). The female resident will encounter resistance and hostility if she calls attention to her different role and needs as a wife and mother.

3. *Physiologic stress.* Residencies tend to be a time of physiologic stress related to loss of sleep and heavy work schedules (Klebanoff et al 1990; Potter 1983). It can be difficult to sustain the stress of a pregnancy physiologically at the same time as experiencing the stress of late nights and missed sleep and meals. One also must consider the impact of such stresses on the unborn child (Kaplan 1970).

4. *Mental stress.* Sleep-deprived interns feel increased sadness and decreased vigor and social affection (Freidman et al 1971). Numerous psychopathologic symptoms can develop, and interns judge themselves to have abnormalities in cognitive, perceptual, and physiologic areas of function (Freidman et al 1971). Finding the mental attention to focus on a child can be difficult.

5. *Difficulty finding child care arrangements.* Because of the erratic and extended schedules of residents, it can be difficult to find appropriate and financially feasible child care arrangements. If the spouse is also a physician or resident, problems can be compounded by overlapping night call schedules.

6. *Difficulties with breast-feeding.* The more erratic the schedule and the less time taken off after delivery, the more difficult it can be to breast-feed an infant. Although breast-feeding problems may occur at any time, residency is the time period in a woman physician's life that can be the worst. Consistent with this, Osborn et al (1990) found that women residents breast-fed for substantially shorter periods of time than wives of men residents.

7. *Discouragement.* Similarly to medical schools, many residencies actively discourage residents from having children.

Overall, the first year of residency is probably the worst time for a woman physician to have children.

## Childbearing During Practice

### Pros

1. *Professional Stature.* Within a few years of finishing the residency, one is more professionally established. One's path is clearer, many professional connections have been made, and colleagues have learned the women physician's professional commitment.

2. *Control.* Control is the biggest advantage of having a child during the practice years. A woman has very little control over her schedule during the training years. However, once out of residency, she can choose her professional situation and she has the option of choosing a situation with flexibility in scheduling.

3. *Affordability.* As practicing physicians earn more money, it is easier to afford children. Child care options are greater when there is money to pay for them.

4. *Matured personality.* The personality of the woman physician will have matured more completely, and the role of physician will be better established. The woman is more certain of herself as a human being and potential mother (Bluestone 1965). One has had more time to evaluate the fantasies and practicalities of motherhood.

5. *Stable partner relationship.* The relationship with a partner is usually more stable and established with additional years together, providing a more secure base for children.

### Cons

1. *Fertility limitations.* Those who delay childbirth in order to complete training feel the pressure of the biological time clock. The number of children one can conceive in a given period of time is limited. Fertility peaks in the early twenties and is on the decline in the thirties, although it does not decline significantly until the late thirties or early forties (Bluestone 1965). Although there are increasing options to enhance fertility, there is no guarantee.

2. *Congenital anomalies.* After 30, the chances of abnormalities in children begin to rise and increase with every passing year. Down syndrome occurs in one in 885 births at the age of 30, one in 365 births at 35, one in 287 births at 36 (Bluestone 1965), and one in 176 at 39.

3. *Maternal and fetal morbidity and mortality.* Older women face a somewhat greater chance of death from childbirth than younger mothers. According to the Centers for Disease Control, there are seven maternal deaths for every 100,000 women ages 20 to 25, as compared to 44 deaths for every 100,000 women in women over the age of 35. Women pregnant for the first time over age 35 have an especially high rate of perinatal death (Bluestone 1965).

4. *Less time for career.* Having children generally means less time for a career. In practice, this may mean less money and perhaps less prestige. In

academic medicine, it may mean slower (or no) promotion. Building professional networks and volunteering for professional activities can take considerable time, often including time away from home. These sorts of activities may seem the most dispensable but may be essential to high level professional advancement.

## Discussion

This summary of the pros and cons of the various times to have children underestimates at least two important factors: the fears inherent in delaying childbirth, and the emotional impact of having children.

Career women such as female physicians often delay having children until they are more established in their careers, such as during or after residency. Fertility decreases as a woman gets older. For this reason, a woman physician typically fears the impact of aging on childbearing ability. What happens if she significantly delays childbearing then cannot get pregnant? Will she and her partner be able to accept this, or will the guilt of believing that she might have been able to get pregnant if she had only tried earlier be overwhelming? Is she tempting fate, risking losing the experience of bearing children, by waiting? Whether or not this is physiologically true, the fear is real and may well be a reason that many women physicians do not delay even longer.

One should also consider the emotional impact of childbirth when deciding at what stage in one's career to have children. Women may have unanticipated feelings of contentment upon the birth of a child (Ordway 1980). The child may stimulate a stronger sense of attachment and pleasure than the mother had expected. Children can be very enticing and fun, but the professional woman may think this will not apply to her to the same extent as to the general public. When the child arrives, and the woman experiences a great amount of contentment and pleasure with the child, the career suddenly may diminish in importance. Some women have children and then quit work, even when they had not originally planned to do so. The woman physician often thinks this will not happen to her. When the child arrives, if the mother has stronger bonding and attachment than expected, she must deal with reprioritizing the child and her career. Should this happen during a time when she feels few or no options in her work situation, she may feel even more guilt. Women should realize the possibility of unanticipated contentment and consider it during planning.

## Financial and Personal

### Maternity Leave

Leaving a newborn child to be cared for by another is an extremely individual decision, and each woman (and potentially her partner) may not be able to identify her own personal needs until after the child is born. Physiologically, many women can return to work fairly quickly after having a child, although a very heavy schedule may be hard to maintain, and those who have C-sections may require additional time to recuperate. Emotionally, though, the best time to return to work is quite variable. Because of the uniqueness of the needs involved, each physician will have to determine their own leave time.

The Federal Pregnancy Discrimination Act of 1978 forbids an employer from discriminating against pregnant employees. The law does not state that a certain amount of maternity leave must be granted, but it does state that if a sick leave exists, that maternity leave must be equal. Most other industrialized nations provide a minimum of 12 weeks of leave (Sayres 1986).

In 1989, one in five medical schools had no written guidelines for maternity leave for faculty physicians, and about half considered maternity leave a form of sick or disability leave (Grisso et al 1991). Although 72% made some allowance in the tenure probationary period for extended leaves of absence, there were few specific provisions to help with childbearing or child rearing.

The U.S. Family and Medical Leave Act of 1993 says that if you have worked for the same company for at least 12 months, have worked at least 1,250 hours in the past year, and work for a company with at least 50 employees within 75 miles of your work site, then you are entitled to take a total of 12 weeks off work without pay, keep any health insurance you already had during the time you are off, and get your old job back, or a job with equal pay, status, and benefits when you return. You can take time for prenatal care, pregnancy illness, or recovery from childbirth. The benefit applies to adoption or foster care placement as well. The time can be used to care for a sick child or relative. You must give 30 days' notice to use the Family and Medical Leave Act. To get help, contact the Women's Bureau of the U.S. Department of Labor (1-800-827-5335) or the Office of Federal Contract Compliance Programs, Employment Standards Administration of the U.S. Department of Labor, Washington, DC 20210 (1-202-219-9475).

The time taken for childbearing is a highly individualized issue. There are abundant stories in female medical circles of women delivering over Thanksgiving vacation and being back in class or at work the following Monday. Although this is uncommon, and many would find it undesirable, in Sinal et al's (1988) study, 60% of women physicians took leaves of 6 weeks or less. About one in five took 7 weeks to 3 months. Klebanoff et al (1990) found the average woman resident worked until the day of or the day before delivery.

## Children Without Childbearing

Adoption is an option for those who so desire, either for infertility or preference. Adoption reduces the physiologic demands on the woman's body and removes some uncertainties. However, other uncertainties are introduced, especially depending on the birth parents of the child and the age of the child. A potential resource is Adoptive Families of America (333 Highway 100 North, Minneapolis, MN 55422, 612-535-4829).

## Choosing To Have No Children

Children are not necessary for a long, fulfilled, and happy life. However, the expectations are so great that women will have children that some women who do not have children feel discriminated against and believe that others wonder "what is wrong" or presume homosexuality. For further discussion, see Elizabeth Whelan's *A Baby . . . Maybe? A Guide to Making the Most Fateful Decision of Your Life.* MacMillan Publishing Company 1975 NY NY

## Raising Children

Even today, as society changes its attitudes toward whom can provide child care, the husband of a woman physician who assumes responsibility for child care is still uncommon (Warde et al 1999), particularly if the husband is also a physician (Sobecks et al 1999; Tesch et al 1992). American Medical Association (1991) data indicate that although 45% of men physicians are married to spouses who work outside the home, 93% of women physicians have spouses who work outside the home. Women physicians spend more time on child care than men physicians (Carr et al 1998). The intent to share child care is often high before pregnancy, but once a child is born, child care is usually the responsibility of the woman, even if the male partner "helps out." One of the major concerns of young women physicians is how to integrate career and family, particularly children. In one study of nonphysician dual-income families, husbands are more likely to share substantial amounts of child care if the first-born child is a boy, the husband and wife work similar numbers of hours, the husband and wife have similar levels of income, and the wives and husbands described the relationship as egalitarian and the division of other labor in the household satisfactory (Fish et al 1992).

There are no easy solutions to combining a career and family life, but the woman physician should know her options, including the cost both monetarily and personally for surrogate care of the children. It may seem obvious, but identifying a mate whose dedication to egalitarianism is evident before having children may increase the likelihood of egalitarian child-rearing practices. It is our experience that many female medical students and young physicians may not believe that such arrangements are possible, although it is also our experience that such arrangements are indeed possible.

### Vignette

Taking James and Elizabeth to meetings was a natural choice, I never questioned it. I'm their mom, and I had a job to do. I want them to grow up knowing it is important to be involved. I really wish more women would be involved and take their children.

*Mary E. LaPlante*

Hints on taking children to meetings

Choose meetings in cities where you have family members who'd like to see/take care of your child for part of the time

Choose meetings with activities scheduled for kids

Take along your spouse, nanny, or other relative

Take along a friend who likes that city & would be willing to do some child care in exchange for hotel housing

Invite a pre-medical or medical student—in exchange for some child care, you can house them (& pay them), pay for their (usually inexpensive) registration, & they can attend some of the meeting, too

Hire a hotel baby sitter or some of the professional organization's staff to take care of your child

Consider taking a cell phone, walkie talkie, or beeper to enhance contact and communication

(by Erica Frank)

## Current Use of Child Care

Nationally, women with children under the age of 5 used relatives (including the father) 41%, organized child care facilities 30%, and family day care settings 17% of the time (Casper 1995). The average weekly cost in 1993 for children of college-educated women was about $93 for each child, including all types of child care used, with greater expense in metropolitan areas and the northeast United States. Day care, one form of child care, cost about $65 per week in 1993.

## Federal Tax Relief

Although a woman physician with children cannot be professionally productive without the support of child care services, the true cost of such services is not tax deductible. There is a little bit of tax relief available to some individuals, however. The Child and Dependent Care Tax Credit became a benefit in 1976 and was increased as part of the 1981 Economic Recovery Tax Act. The credit decreases with increasing income, and this tax credit is more likely to help students and residents than practicing physicians. To claim this tax credit, the physician employer must provide the name and social security number of the child care provider. Some employers also offer a dependent care flexible benefit plan, where a set amount of money is set aside for the year and spent out of pretax dollars. This is helpful, but once the amount of money is determined it cannot be changed; if the amount was overestimated, the money placed in the account is forfeited at the end of the year. There are also rules on what is considered eligible, and it does not cover all of the types of costs that are incurred.

## Choosing Child Care Services

The people that a woman physician hires to provide child care or other household help are critical to her. The effort and care taken to select reliable, warm, interested, appropriately stimulating and honest people will be invaluable. It is wise to choose individuals who use child-rearing techniques and standards similar to the parents. This will ease the physician's worries about her family and provide her the physical and mental freedom to pursue her career.

There is no guarantee of quality in child care services. Some states regulate day care facilities, but fewer regulate the small group care setting out of someone's home. Enforcement is highly variable.

Plenty of time is needed to find child care. A minimum of 4 to 6 weeks is suggested. If this length of time coincides with the time taken off for maternity leave, the decision may be made to wait until the child is born to hunt for child care. Some women are uncomfortable with not having arrangements made before the child is born, and some locations (such as competitive child care facilities) have long waiting lists, so earlier searching may be required. Many facilities will not take reservations. If a person is hired to come into the home, an additional 2 weeks should be added, because this process takes longer, and it is reasonable to hire the individual before he or she is actually required (i.e., in advance of delivery).

> One resource is the Family Resource Handbook, Presidents and Fellows of Harvard College, 1998, 617-432-1615. Another is the National Association of Child Care Resource and Referral Agencies, PO Box 402-46, Washington, DC 20016 1-800-424-2246 or 202-333-4194.

Particularly problematic aspects of caring for children often include how to have kids taken care of before school, after school activities that involve transportation, ill children, special needs children, and care during night call when the parents are unavailable.

Below is a listing of the common types of arrangements in order of least to most expensive (by typical cost) with their advantages and disadvantages. Many woman physicians end up using more than one type of arrangement.

## Care by a Family Member

The husband or partner of some women physicians care for the children. Most would consider this the most ideal arrangement. Backup arrangements for illness are needed. Alternatively, another family member may provide a portion or all of the child care for a woman physician.

### Advantages

1. The physician and child usually knows the caregiver quite well.
2. Depending on arrangements, this may be less costly than other alternatives, and, if not, the money stays in the family.

3. The caregiver may be familiar with and understand the extent of the parents' commitment to certain principles.

4. Sustainable, lasting affection is promoted between the child and her/his relative.

5. The caregiver is particularly invested in the child's best interests.

6. A relative may be flexible with hours, helping with overnight stays, night call, or other evening child care needs.

### Disadvantages

1. Differences in child-rearing views may be more difficult to discuss with someone in the family.

2. Financial issues may be less clear.

3. There is dependence on one individual.

Many women physicians who utilize family members for regular child care pay for the services.

## Day-Care Centers

Day-care centers tend to be an unpopular choice for child care for women physicians (Sinal et al 1988). However, they sometimes are the best choice.

### Advantages

1. They are usually the least expensive formal alternative.

2. They may be regulated.

3. There is no reliance on one specific provider (which helps if the child care provider gets sick, for example).

4. They are readily available.

5. They frequently have educational programs for the children.

6. Children have the opportunity to socially interact with other children their own age.

### Disadvantages

1. They have set hours of operation, which often do not coincide with the work hours of physicians.

2. Some will not accept infants.

3. There are large numbers of children with relatively few caregivers. As a result, there is less individual attention for each child.

4. The large number of children in a close environment leads to the spread of infection (such as giardia and respiratory infections), and has been postulated to be associated with the development of resistant organisms, such as found increasingly with otitis media (ear infections).

5. They are inflexible in their arrangements.

6. Very few will care for ill children.

7. The parent may be asked to participate in administrative activities.

## Child Care in Someone Else's Home

*Advantages*

1. Frequently the home is in a convenient location near the physician's home.

2. This arrangement tends to be more flexible than day-care centers.

3. There are fewer children than in day-care centers.

4. Some will care for ill children.

*Disadvantages*

1. There is usually reliance on one individual.

2. The arrangement may be unregulated.

Finding a local home care provider usually means seeking out information through the grapevine, such as through neighbors, a local church, or school teachers. States that require licensing will have a list of licensed providers.

## Child Care in the Physician's Home

*Advantages*

1. This type of care is the most convenient; children are with their possessions and food and do not need to be dressed and prepared for child care outside the home.

2. There is a higher likelihood the caregiver will care for a moderately ill child.

3. There is more likely to be flexibility of hours.

4. Some caregivers can transport children to activities before or after school.

5. Some caregivers may also do housework.

*Disadvantages*

1. It is more expensive.

2. There is heavy reliance on one individual's availability, promptness, and reliability.

3. There is less privacy and security of the home.

4. The physician must follow federal rules concerning taxes and workers' compensation (see sidebar).

5. The physician may also need to provide other common employment benefits, such as health care insurance.

6. The physician may need to provide a car for transporting the children.

Employer Requirements:

*Employer identification numbers.* You will need a federal employer number available from the Internal Revenue Service (Form SS-4; call 1-800-TAX-FORM) and a state employer number.

*State and federal unemployment tax.* The rate is set by the state and paid to the state, although not all states require an unemployment tax. The federal unemployment insurance is usually paid annually and can be paid with your annual tax return. The amount paid to the federal government depends on the amount paid to the state, and there is a specific IRS form to complete (Schedule H). Payment is required on domestic wages of $1,000 or more a calendar quarter.

*Social Security and Medicare taxes.* Social Security and Medicare taxes must be paid if a private household employee is paid more than $1,000 in a year, except when the worker is a spouse, a child under age 21, or a parent working in the home (use Form 942 for the parent in the home). The Social Security tax is equal to 12.4% of income up to $65,400, which the employer and employee can split 50/50 or the employer can elect to pay all of it. The Medicare tax is 1.45% for both the employer and the employee. These taxes can be paid with the employer's annual federal income tax return.

*Federal and state income taxes.* With a single employee, the employer can either withhold federal income taxes (Form W-4, Employees Withholding Allowance Certificate; see IRS Publication 15, Circular E, Employer's Tax Guide for Withholding Tables) or agree with the employee that the employee will file quarterly income tax statements. Similar mechanism is used for state taxes.

*Workers' Compensation Insurance.* This is usually handled by a local insurance company and is usually experience-rated.

*Annual W-2 Forms.* The employer is required to complete and submit W-2 and W-3 forms to the employee, the Social Security Administration, and the state government by January 31 of each year for any employee for whom income, Social Security, or Medicare taxes have been withheld or to whom an earned income credit has been paid in advance.

*Minimum wage.* Under the Fair Labor Standards Act, the minimum wage laws must be followed for domestic workers, and the current minimum wage is $5.15 as of September 1997; some states have higher minimum wages. Hours in excess of 40 hours a week must be paid at 1½ times the minimum wage unless the employee resides in the household. No premium pay is required for holidays or weekends. There are no required rest periods, discharge notices, or severance pay.

See your accountant for more details.

## Live-Ins/Au Pairs

Live-in arrangements are both the most convenient and the most expensive type of in-home care. Adequate living space must be available, and the privacy issues are magnified. The amount of salary may be slightly less, because room and board is being provided. Au-pair arrangements are a mechanism whereby international young women and men of college age can live and help with child care in the home in the United States. Au pairs are usually arranged through an agency, and there are specific rules, such as the hours the individual can work, and the length of time the au pair can stay in the United States. A perceived disadvantage of the au-pair arrangement is that the individuals are here for a limited time; one specific advantage is the potential for introduction of the family to another culture.

## Other Arrangements

**Other types of arrangements** that are often used include the following:

Extended school days (before or after) are available in many school districts or may be provided by a local Young Men's/Women's Christian Association (YMCA/YWCA) or day-care center.

Local college, graduate, or medical students may be available for overnight stays or to provide child transportation.

Neighborhood adolescents may be available for babysitting.

Some services provide after-school transportation (getting to be more common in large suburban areas).

Local child car-pooling arrangements are common.

Co-op arrangements can be made with other parents.

## Assuring Quality Child Care

No matter which child care arrangement is made, the parents will want to assure that it is high-quality care. Here are some general suggestions:

Review in advance the caregiver's child care beliefs, such as discipline and feeding practices.

Visit unexpectedly.

Consider getting an individual provider bonded (contact the state board of health).

Treat child care providers with respect and value their opinions and ideas.

Give holiday gifts and birthday cards, including from your children.

Praise your childcare provider at appropriate times; show appreciation.

Regular, ongoing communication is essential.

In recent years, technology has also become available to help parents. Some day-care centers offer videotaping that can be viewed through the Internet throughout the day. Some parents have placed hidden microphones and cameras in their homes, occasionally detecting child neglect and even child abuse. This is usually done when there is a high level of suspicion of problems. In general, if you have a high level of suspicion, it is probably wise to fire the employee.

If a good employee has proven her/himself, but you will no longer be their employer, consider placing an ad to help them find a job ("nanny employer seeking new placement") or finding someone you know who needs a similar employee.

## Care After School

When the child begins school, arrangements for child care change. They must now encompass the new problem of transportation to and from school plus care before and after school hours. If the physician has a live-in or come-in housekeeper, this should be included in her/his job description and special attention paid to car availability.

For those who are not so fortunate, special arrangements must be made for transportation. If the school bus transports children to and from the neighborhood, you may wish to use it (in spite of children's protests). But alternative arrangements must be made for missed buses or outside activities that end after the last bus (some school systems have special activity buses). If the physician relies heavily on a neighbor or other individual for transportation of her children, she should consider payment or some reciprocal service for the time, effort, and cost.

Some schools and child care centers offer after-school arrangements. Some child care centers send buses to schools to transport children to the day-care center. Similar arrangements can be made with a trusted neighbor, family member, or paid employee. Neighborhood teens might be interested in the job, but may be less reliable because of their own after-school activities and their age.

There are many latchkey children in the United States, i.e., those who go home to an empty house and stay there alone until the parent arrives home from work, but it is not an option chosen by many women physicians. This arrangement works best for mature and responsible children who have activities outlined for them and ready access to their parent, usually through a telephone. Parents should regularly call. Four studies since 1982 have found no differences in outcomes between latchkey children and children cared for by an adult in the home (Zylke 1988). However, being removed from adult supervision may make an adolescent more susceptible to peer pressure (Zylke 1988).

## Child Care During the Summer

Figuring out what to do with school-age children during the summer can be perplexing. Some large day-care centers or sports clubs offer summer programs including day camps, frequent field trips, swimming lessons, and structured outside games. YMCAs and YWCAs also provide many activities. The local recreation department can often be of assistance. Some churches offer special programs as well. Unfortunately, summer programs are not as prevalent as most working women would like, and the ideal program may not be available in a location convenient for transportation. Another method of summer child care is to hire a responsible teenager or college student to babysit for the summer.

## Guidelines for Hiring a Care Provider in the Home

There are two basic choices. The physician can hire through an employment agency or directly as an employer, whether or not the individual hired has been found with the help of a referral agency. Hiring through an employment agency may result in finding an individual more quickly who has already been prescreened. Employment agencies are the employer, and thus take care of the various taxes and insurance required. Some agencies provide a backup in case of illness of the provider. Some physicians have had excellent experience with agencies, and others have not. There is usually a significant agency fee. The fee can be avoided by hiring directly as an employer.

These steps outlined below apply to both live-ins as well as other providers who will be coming into the home when the physician is acting directly as the employer.

1. Prepare a list of qualifications needed.

2. Develop an application form (consider one from the physician's office practice).

3. Post the notice in the city paper, a neighborhood paper, or in churches. Describe the job available and the minimum requirements. Network by telling friends, fellow church members, and coworkers of job availability. Consider using a post office box number rather than giving out a home phone number and address.

4. Ask all applicants to send a résumé, then screen for whom you wish to complete an application and consider for interview.

5. Call all references or ask for written letters of reference. Telephone calls tend to yield more negative information. Estimates are that half of the references will be bogus, and calling can help detect some of these.

6. Interview candidates. Consider doing this at the candidate's home, or in the formality of the physician office. Have a list of questions ready, including such items as discipline, child stimulation and activities, dietary habits, smoking, alcohol and drug use, use of car seats, vacations, and ownership of a car. Provide sample situations and ask how the care provider would handle them.

7. Before hiring, be sure that the potential employee is eligible by completing the Department of Labor Immigration and Naturalization Service Form I-9. See *http://www.dol.gov/dol*. The employee must have a Social Security number (available by calling 1-800-SSA-1213).

8. Agree to regularly evaluate the employee and provide appropriate compensation. The possibility that the employee will need to be fired some day must be considered. A probationary period should be considered. The caregiver should be fired if he or she is not meeting expectations. It is more difficult to deal with inadequate child care and irresponsibility on a day-to-day basis that it is to fire a person or find a replacement.

9. Provide a written job description (Table 6-1).

TABLE 6-1.
SAMPLE JOB DESCRIPTION FOR THE SMITH-JONES FAMILY HELPER

The job includes:
1. Child care: Complete care of the baby in our absence. This is the top priority. No other responsibility or personal need is to interfere with this.
   a. We follow general discipline measures.
   b. We expect regular stimulation, such as reading and interactive activities, for most of the baby's waking time during the day.
2. Routine house cleaning: Make beds; change sheets every week. Dust furniture, scrub and wax floors, vacuum carpets, clean bathrooms, and wash dishes.
   a. Clean stove, refrigerator, and dishwasher once a month and as needed.
   b. Wash windows twice a year and as needed.
   c. Clean and dust closets and cupboards twice a year and as needed.
3. Laundry.
4. Ironing of the few items that require it.
5. Start supper (food and menus will be provided).
6. Miscellaneous light errands (e.g., pick up dry cleaning).
7. Other duties as given by Drs. Jones or Smith.

Work begins July 25; the baby is due July 1.

Hours: 7:30 A.M. to 5:00 to 6:00 P.M., when one parent arrives home.
   One Saturday morning a month 7:30 A.M. to 2:00 P.M.
   Not on most Thursdays (schedule will be provided).
   One-half the office holidays (when Dr. Jones is on call).

Personal days off: Two weeks a year with 4-week advance notice. We prefer to try to arrange vacation schedules together in advance. We may arrange to have you go on an occasional vacation with us to help with child care.

Job evaluation: First one at 1 month, then at 3 months, then every 6 months with raise consideration every year.

I have received a copy of the job description and have reviewed and read the listed responsibilities with Dr. Jones.


_____     _____
      Applicant Name                   Date


## The Effect of Surrogate Care on Children

The American tradition of the mother staying at home raising the child may create feelings of pride or of guilt and inadequacy in those who do not. It is, however, a distinctly American tradition that is no longer the norm. Years ago, other countries developed day-care centers and domestic helpers much more extensively.

Physicians are not taught much about mother and infant attachment (Potter 1983). Intuitively, it is felt that the mother and infant interaction in child rearing is paramount. Freud produced guilt in mothers in the 1920s by espousing the belief that mothers were considered to be almost fully responsible for the emotional and psychological well-being of their children. This was reinforced by Benjamin Spock in the 1950s when he wrote about the importance of the mother's presence in meeting a child's emotional needs (Scott 1978). It now seems a rather formidable task, and probably unnecessary, to feel solely responsible for the psychological development of any person. Some physicians who are not full-time parents may take particular joy in the time they do spend with their children and approach even mundane child rearing with special pleasure.

A recent longitudinal study on the effects of early child care supported by the National Institute of Child Health and Human Development found that quality child care, defined as positive caregiving and language stimulation given in the child care environment, is directly related to early cognitive and language development. Other major predictors of children's cognitive and linguistic outcomes included family income, maternal vocabulary, home environment, and maternal cognitive stimulation. This study involved more than 1,300 families and their children, standardized tests, such as the Bayley Scales of Infant Development, and videotaped interactions of the mother and child. The children were enrolled before 1 month of age and followed to age 7. (This information is from the National Institute of Child Health and Human Development Web site, *http://www.hig.gov/news/pr/apr97/nichd-03.htm*, and the press release of April 3, 1997.) Thus, it is important to have good-quality child care, but the study found that most child care was of good quality.

### Health of Physicians' Children

There is little information on the health of physicians' children. It is of interest that, in general, physicians tend to take their children to the doctor at later stages in an illness than do other parents (Wasserman et al 1989). The children also tend to be referred to specialists directly by their parents. There is also less documentation of a psychosocial history in the chart of a physician's child. In a study of adolescent children of physicians presenting for psychiatric help, no typical syndrome could be identified (Stein and Leventhal 1984).

## SUMMARY

Life is full of choices, and few are larger than deciding whether, when, and how to have and raise children. This is compounded for someone pursuing a profession, particularly one that has many demands and rewards similar to motherhood. Most women physicians do have children, and must consider many factors in deciding when to have the children. For those who do have children, the demands and frustrations, as well as rewards, can be great.

Child care will continue to be one of the biggest challenges that a woman physician has to address. The appropriate child care that best fits the parents and the working situation should be chosen, but will change over time. Effective child care permits the woman physician the freedom to pursue her career more actively. Although the woman physician may feel guilty about surrogate child care, children have been shown to be capable of developing multiple attachments without harm. There seems to be a positive relationship between working mothers and high achievement of the children. New options for dealing with difficult child care issues may develop as more and more women enter the work force.

## CHAPTER 7

# Sexual Harassment and Sex Discrimination

Marjorie A. Bowman

For women physicians, sexual harassment and sex discrimination are still distressingly common. Sexual harassment also happens to men physicians.

Sexual harassment and sex discrimination are different but related. They have different definitions and seemingly different perpetrators. The U.S. Equal Employment Opportunity Commission notes that sexual harassment is a form of sex discrimination. Both are violations of Title VII of the Civil Rights Act of 1964. Some actions may also violate the Violence Against Women Act of 1994 or individual state laws.

The event(s) may be minor or major. Women physicians should consider what their response should be—how to respond immediately, and whether or not administrative or legal redress should be pursued.

## DEFINITIONS

With sexual harassment, the individual experiencing it helps to define it—the essential term utilized is "unwanted." Usually, sexual harassment is separated into two types: quid pro quo (a person's submission or rejection of sexual advances is used in employment decisions) or hostile environment. The adverse consequence can be solely that the woman feels the environment is inimical. Generally, quid pro quo harassment may require only one incident, but a hostile environment requires repetition to be considered harassment. No economic injury is required, and the harassment may be to someone else, but create a problematic work environment.

Generally, physical harassment (touching) has been more readily identified and condemned than verbal harassment, partly because of the ubiquitous nature of verbal harassment and the difficulties with definition. For example, when is flirtation harassment? A furtive look? Legally, verbal remarks and actions are harassment when they are unwanted and create a hostile work environment or adverse employment decisions, but on a day-to-day basis many people are unsure. Because of these uncertainties, there is a stated fear of the development of intimate relationships from a work environment, yet many such relationships do develop and may flourish without any harassment occurring or charges being filed.

---

*Steven Jeffes argues that appearance discrimination (discriminating on whether or not someone is good looking) pervades our society and employment interactions* (Appearance Is Everything, *Sterling House, 1998*).

---

Sex discrimination is frequently more difficult to identify than sexual harassment. It may be subtle and is rarely stated. The woman cannot define that she has been discriminated against. The adverse consequences of sex discrimination are described in terms of job outcomes and advancement. This may mean that legally it does not apply to students, but most medical schools take harassment and discrimination seriously. For example, did women applicants, given their backgrounds and capabilities, get ranked as high on the National Resident Matching Program list as the men applicants? Are as many referrals sent to the woman physician as to a similar man? Because of varying backgrounds, it can be difficult to identify the "similar" men and women. In many circumstances, people are more comfortable with other people who are like them, and perpetrators of sex discrimination are often unaware of their own discrimination ("She made me uncomfortable, and I liked him better").

Women earn about three-fourths of what men do in the United States, and are away from their jobs longer. The difference in hourly wage is less dramatic, with women earning about 80% of men's hourly wage. An analysis (Reed 1999) indicated that for men and women starting work at age 21 and working to the end of their 64th year, the lifetime difference becomes dramatic. The man, starting at $30,000 per year, would earn $3,462,386. The woman would start at $22,800 and would earn $2,631,446, a difference of $830,940. If the woman took 5 years away from work (which is average for women), the difference would increase by another $175,770. We do not have the same types of figures for women physicians, but we know that women physicians consistently earn less than men physicians on an hourly or yearly basis. However, as outlined in Chapter 13, some estimates have shown that young female and male physicians earn about the same amount when the figures are adjusted for confounding factors such as practice type and specialty and work hours.

## SEXUAL HARASSMENT AND SEX DISCRIMINATION AND ABUSE IN MEDICINE

Sex harassment is noted by the majority of medical students (Lubitz and Dguyen 1996; Richman et al 1992) and residents (Cook et al 1996; Komaromy et al 1993). At one school, women completing their clerkship year reported three times the rate of sexual abuse as men (64% compared to 21%) (Lubitz and Nguyen 1996). Nine times as many female as male graduating medical students reported "unwanted sexual advances by school personnel" (Bickel and Ruffin 1995) (12.6% versus 1.4%). Sexual harassment is not just from supervisors. Almost half of the sexual harassment incidents reported by the women students on internal medicine clerkships from 11 medical schools involved patients, and most were inappropriate remarks or refusal to see the student based on their sex (Elnicki et al 1999). A few women were inappropriately touched by patients.

The reported rates of harassment/abuse/discrimination in different studies vary substantially, primarily because of the wording of the surveys. Women physicians are less likely to report "sexual harassment" than "unwanted sexual attention," apparently not defining some of the unwanted sexual attention as harassment (Lenhart et al 1991). Schiffman and Frank (1995) review likely reasons for this, including that (1) many women cope with harassment by refusing to acknowledge its existence or seriousness; (2) the term *sexual harassment* seems too formal for such an everyday event; and, unfortunately, (3) sexual harassment is accepted from early childhood on into adult life.

Other types of abuse are common. Belittlement was the most common type reported in one study (Elnicki et al 1999). Public humiliation and someone else taking credit for one's work were commonly mentioned in one study (Baldwin et al 1991). Psychological abuse and physical abuse from patients and families are common (Cook et al 1996). One in five residents reported being physically assaulted (Cook et al 1996).

In medical residencies, women residents noted sex harassment more often than men (about 3:1, 75% compared to 25%) in the Komaromy et al (1993) study; in the study by Cook et al (1996), over 90% of all respondents reported sexist jokes. The perpetrators reported by the women were more likely of higher status, i.e., attending physicians, than reported by the men, i.e., nurses, and thus the women felt there was a greater negative effect of the harassment (Komaromy et al 1993). Gay, lesbian, and bisexual physicians report more lifestyle harassment but not sexual harassment (Brogan et al 1999) than other women physicians.

## Vignette

Have your successes ever threatened your boss? When you assert your ideas, are you labeled "pushy" or "controlling"? Does your mentor consider you ungrateful if you challenge his advice? Are you perceived as angry when you do not smile? Women's careers are frequently derailed or slowed because men with power over them have so little experience with goal-oriented women in the workplace (generous interpretation).

When such questions arise in a significant relationship, the earlier you can diagnose and treat the pathology, the better. Is it a pattern (e.g., does he have problems with other strong women)? If not, is it something about your style or the messages you're sending that you need to work on? If his trouble with you is repeated in other relationships, the cause may be sexual insecurity (unconscious = unreachable). If so, start strategizing now to put as much distance between you as possible. If he appears educable (e.g., behaviors stemming from a well-meant paternalism), can you (or an ally) motivate him to examine the negative consequences of his gender stereotypes? If yes, might he become an ally? (Tip: look for every opportunity to mentor and support male colleagues who are closet feminists). If the problem is a Queen Bee (i.e., a woman threatened by other women's successes), substitute pronouns—although here the insecurity is more likely to be of the chronic, situational type.

Can we more consciously be creating workplaces and homes where roles and relationships are unhampered by gender stereotypes?

*Janet Bickel, experienced speaker/writer*
*on issues about women in medicine.*

As compared to women in residency, U.S. women physicians in practice report less harassment (25% report gender-based and 11% sexual harassment) (Frank et al 1998). In a study of women physicians in Massachusetts, about a quarter reported sexual harassment and a half reported some form of sex discrimination (Lenhart et al 1991). Among women faculty throughout the United States, 47% of the younger women and 70% of the older women but fewer than one-third of men faculty reported gender-based discrimination (Carr et al 2000). Few men faculty (<3%) reported the more substantial harassment experienced by about one-third of women faculty. Primary care physicians reported less, and surgical physicians more, gender-based discrimination. Interestingly, in this study more women (31%) than men (11%) also had felt advantaged by their gender.

In the study of Massachusetts women physicians, women who were younger, unmarried, and in settings with more men were more likely to report harassment; this is similar to studies of women other than physicians (Lenhart et al 1991). In the Women Physicians' Health Study, certain characteristics were associated with the report of ever having been subjected to gender-based harassment: women physicians who were divorced or separated, not Asian or "other" race, those specializing in historically male specialties, those identifying themselves as politically more liberal, and those not living in the eastern United States. Similar to the medical students, women physicians in practice also report sexual harassment by patients (Phillips and Schneider 1993; Schneider and Phillips 1997).

---

*Although sexual contact between patients and physicians is not governed by employment law, it is unethical and can easily lead to the loss of the physician's medical license (Gartrell et al 1992).*

---

## DISCRIMINATION BY PATIENTS

Some patients also discriminate, although not by legal definitions. Some patients prefer not to see women physicians (Engleman 1974; Haar et al 1975; Kasteler and Humle 1980; Needle and Murray 1977). Others prefer to see women physicians, particularly women who are more androgynous (Weyrauch et al 1990) as compared to highly masculine or feminine. Among adolescents, both female adolescent contraceptive patients (Philliber and Jones 1982) and male adolescents for genital exams (Van Ness and Lynch 2000), preferred female physicians. The preference for female physicians was particularly strong among African-American male adolescents. A substantial minority of patients report they do not want to see gay/bisexual/lesbian physicians (Druzin et al 1998). Overall, the effect of the patient preferences is that women physicians have a higher percentage of women patients in their practices than do men physicians (Bensing et al 1993; Challacombe 1983; Hartzema and Christensen 1983).

---

*Female physicians see more female patients than do male physicians.*

---

Earlier research (Engleman 1974) found that patients generally preferred male doctors and believed female doctors were less competent and experienced. However, patients who had seen women physicians were more positive toward them. This suggests that as more women have entered medicine, the concerns about competence and experience have probably decreased, which is consistent with current facts and figures on medical practice.

The gender of the physician appears to be more important for certain types of exams or complaints. For example, Petravage et al (1979) found about one-fifth of her sample specifically preferred women physicians for breast and pelvic exams. Ackerman-Ross and Sochat (1980) similarly found that certain types of complaints predicted preference for same-sex physician, particularly sexual dysfunction, followed by physical examination, and blood in urine, with no difference by sex of the physician for sore throat. However, the authors found a general preference for same-sex physician, with men more strongly shifting to wanting male physicians for more intimate problems than female patients to female physicians. Also, of importance to understanding this literature, patients were more likely to choose a physician of their sex who was more highly recommended by others; recommendation by others was more important than the sex of the physician in determining which physician the patient selected.

As a result of patient choices, female physicians see different kinds of problems: more family planning, female genital problems, social problems, and endocrine/metabolic problems but fewer male genital and musculoskeletal problems (Bensing et al 1993). Interestingly, in the Bensing et al study, the female physicians also saw more social problems and endocrine/metabolic problems in male as well as female patients.

In general, patients may be more satisfied when they have the opportunity to choose their own physician, thus being able to choose one with the characteristics desired, whether or not one of the important aspects of choice is the sex of the physician. When not able to choose the physicians, the patients may generally be less satisfied, particularly with physicians with nonnormative characteristics, such as physicians who are women or black (Ross et al 1982).

---

*There is selectivity on the part of patients for the sex of the physician, dependent on circumstances, the type of problem, and expectations.*

---

## EFFECTS OF SEXUAL HARASSMENT AND SEX DISCRIMINATION

The outcomes of these abhorrent behaviors are not fully known. In nonphysician studies, psychological distress is common and about 1 in 10 women report changing jobs because of sexual harassment. Reports of harassment by medical students have been associated with poorer psychological outcomes (Lubitz and Nguyen 1996; Richman et al 1992), and self-reported lower self-confidence, lower self-esteem, and impaired ability to learn (Lubitz and Nguyen 1996). Women faculty (Carr et al 2000) who experienced gender-based discrimination reported slightly lower career satisfaction and professional confidence than, but had similar numbers of publications to, other women faculty. We also know that practicing women physicians with histories of depression or suicide attempts were more likely to report having been harassed (Frank et al 1998)—was the depression related to the harassment, or did the depression make women more at risk for harassment or the perception of harassment? (Perhaps all are true.) Women physicians who felt more in control in their work environments and were more satisfied with being a physician were less likely to report having been harassed (Frank et al 1998). Once again, the question of which comes first can be asked. Women who have not faced harassment or discrimination may feel more at ease in the profession, or it may be that dissatisfied women are more likely face circumstances they perceive as harassment.

Also, importantly, is the lower confidence level of women (Bickel and Ruffin 1995) (also discussed in Chapter 14) at least partially the result of sexual harassment and sex discrimination? The above literature clearly suggests the answer is a disappointing, disheartening, yes. However, perhaps this means that more emphasis on decreasing the rates of sexual harassment and sex discrimination could yield more confident and mentally healthier women physicians.

## SEXUAL STEREOTYPING AS A FORM OF DISCRIMINATION

One of the subtle forms of discrimination is sexual stereotyping (Conley 1993). In our society, the attributes *assertive, decisive,* and *capable* are considered male. Women who display similar abilities may be thought of as aggressive (a more negative term), pushy, unfeminine, and uncaring. Women leaders providing the same suggestions and arguments are viewed more negatively than men leaders (Butler and Geis 1990). The field of medicine is actually one where both traditional male and female attributes are frequently desired—patients want physicians who are capable and decisive (traditional male), but caring and warm (traditional female). See Chapter 14 for a more detailed description of the literature and a discussion.

U.S. Equal Employment Opportunity Commission definition of sexual harassment: "Unwelcome sexual advances, requests for sexual favors, and other verbal or physical conduct of a sexual nature constitute sexual harassment when submission to or rejection of this conduct explicitly or implicitly affects an individual's employment, unreasonably interferes with an individual's work performance or creates an intimidating, hostile or offensive work environment" (last update January 15, 1997).

### Example 1
During my internship, I was rounding with my otherwise all-male team, tarried to finish up with one of my patients, and ran down the hallway to catch up. My attending yelled down the hall "oh, don't hurry, I'm just enjoying watching the female form in action". I was embarassed, but this was an isolated incident from this otherwise exemplary attending and I pursued no redress.

*(continued)*

(continued)
## Example 2
One evening, also during my internship, I agreed to meet an extremely prominent, trusted mentor who was visiting from out of town. The only time he could meet was at 10, & I agreed to meet him in his hotel lobby. About an hour into our discussion, I came up with a good idea, and he fondled my arm & said "you always stimulate me in so many ways". When I tearfully tried discussing this with him several years later, he said "well, it can't have been too much of a problem, we're still working together." I knew lots of women who had worked this man, and checked with them. They had never heard of this kind of behavior happening with him, & I chose not to pursue it further. Even now, many years after the incident, I am still fearful I will experience negative repercussions from publishing this.

Examples from the lives of the authors.
Sex discrimination: One author and a male physician with similar backgrounds were hired at about the same time and given similar job responsibilities. The author had the opportunity to find out what this man was being paid (she asked, he told), and it was significantly higher than her own income. She confronted their mutual boss, who cited a certain aspect of the male's background that was perceived to be important; she was also told that she would make as much money within a couple of years. The income increase did not happen, and she believes she was discriminated against. Long-term outcome: this boss and the author remain professional acquaintances and friends and occasionally call on each other for work-related items. The author is probably just a little bit financially poorer, but stronger!

Sexual harassment: A male physician in position of authority over one of the authors recurrently mentioned her sexual attractiveness and called her "honey." She felt awkward telling him to stop, often saying nothing and occasionally parrying the comments with "honey?" One day an inappropriate comment about her sexual attractiveness was made in front of the dean, and the dean asked her if this type of comment was what all the women complained about. The answer was obviously yes. The dean said he would speak to the man and apparently did so. After that the comments were toned down, but "honey" continued, always followed by "But I'm not allowed to say that, am I?" Long-term outcome: we suspect he retired still making comments, but they were less blunt, less vulgar, and less frequent. He was not demoted, and we do not think he was ever sued.

Sexual harassment: My supervising resident climbed into my bed when I was a medical student and starting kissing me. I persistently told him that I was not interested, and he went back to his bed (which was unfortunately in the same room as mine!). We continued to "room together" the remainder of the clerkship (it felt like there was no alternative), and
(continued)

*(continued)*

no further incidents occurred. I got a reasonable grade on the clerkship. I did not report him.

Sexual harassment: A married faculty attending from my specialty of choice came to my apartment after my clerkship was over, but before application letters of reference were done. I was stumped as to why he came until he started to fondle my hair and compliment my appearance almost immediately upon coming in the door. When I insisted, he left. I did not report him. Years later, he died suddenly of a heart attack. Rumor was that he was in bed with one of his residents who was not his wife.

## AGE, RACE, SEX, AND NATIONAL ORIGIN DISCRIMINATION AND HARASSMENT

Age, race, sex and national origin are the characteristics generally considered under discrimination or harassment. Both race discrimination and racial harassment have clearly been upheld through the U.S. courts. Age discrimination is protected under the Age Discrimination in Employment Act of 1967 (ADEA; see *http://www.eeoc.gov/facts/age.html*). With this law, individuals who are 40 years of age or older are legally protected from employment discrimination based on age. This law applies to both employees and job applicants. The Older Workers Benefit Protection Act of 1990 amended the ADEA to include prohibition of benefit denial to older employees.

## WHEN THE LAW DOES NOT APPLY

There are limits to the laws, and not everyone is protected legally. The Age Discrimination in Employment Act of 1967 applies only to employers of 20 or more employees, and may not include state and local governments. Title 7 of the Civil Rights Act applies to employers who have at least 15 workers. Congress has traditionally been excluded from all of these legislative acts. Many Americans, including many physicians, work for small employers, and thus the laws do not directly apply to their circumstances. Physicians are often the employers, and thus should know the laws of employment. The laws encourage proper behavior by employers, but do not guarantee it.

## WHAT TO DO?

Sexual harassment in particular is taken much more seriously now than in the past. At the time of the first edition of this book, women had little recourse, and I suspect laughter would have followed reporting some types of behavior, particularly verbal, that are now routinely considered harassment.

What to Do?

1. Follow employer policy.

2. Keep a journal. Write down perceived negative actions, along with steps you have taken.

3. Seek emotional support from friends, family, or support groups.

4. Talk to other women at work and get information on how they have been treated. The National Labor Relations Act protects your right to meet together.

5. Find out your rights and responsibilities. Unions, the Equal Employment Opportunity Commission Web sites (*http://www.eoc*) or local offices (under U.S. Government, EEOC in the phone book), employer handbooks, and state fair employment practices offices are some sources of information. The Women's Bureau Clearinghouse is available at 1-800-827-5335.

6. Continue personally exemplary behavior.

7. Weigh pros and cons to determine your personally selected action.

Sexual harassment policies are required for each work site. If you feel victimized, you should follow the policy, which generally tells you to first tell the harasser to stop. This may be best done in writing, which increases the clarity, helps the woman choose her words, and lets the accused know the seriousness. The second step, which you may follow if you do not feel you can confront the harasser, or if the harasser does not stop the unwanted behavior, is to talk with the person identified in the organization to handle these matters. Witnesses are frequently key (whom should the employer believe?), but are not required by law. Untrue accusations can ruin careers, and true accusations are often not easily proven.

The law requires an employer to have a policy and to attempt to prevent harassment and to stop harassment that is occurring. Thus many institutions have classes or seminars for everyone on sexual harassment, including individuals who are not supervisors. For example, residents can be harassers of nurses but are not their supervisors, creating a hostile work environment, so the residents need to know the limits as well. With the Civil Rights Act of 1991, monetary damages can be assessed when sexual harassment has occurred.

Sex discrimination often requires facts—were all women in a specific job class given lower pay than men in the same job? Facts are often difficult to ascertain, and thus sex discrimination can be tough to prove. Is the lack of advancement, lack of a specific job perk, or whatever, the result of overt or covert discrimination? As happened to one of the authors, employers often have a rationale, even when confronted. Similarly, one of the authors reviewed salaries of men and women faculty for a medical school. It was clear that the women earned less. But the chairs of the respective departments could readily cite reasons that those women earned less: they did not take on-call assignments, they brought in fewer grants, they were not in charge of the clinic (but might have been in charge of the medical student rotation), they did fewer procedures and thus brought lower clinical income to the department, etc. When is it discrimination?

## WHEN TO PURSUE LEGAL RECOURSE

Women residents in one study said they rarely reported sexual harassment, primarily because they thought they would not be helped (Komaromy et al 1993). Men also rarely reported sexual harassment, but because they felt they had dealt with the issue on their own. Similar results were found in the study by Cook et al (1996).

Threatening legal action can bring results. However, there are downsides to the legal route. The legal system frequently takes years. Generally, the complainant is under a shadow of suspicion from fellow workers, and potentially from friends and family, and certainly from potential future employers. (Someone who sued in the past seems more likely to sue again, something employers do not want.) If the facts are clear in support of the woman's position, the employer frequently settles prior to court proceedings; thus it is the less clear cases that are most likely to end up in front of a judge or jury. The press may become involved and the case may receive wide attention. Psychological symptoms are common. Thus, legal recourse should not be undertaken lightly.

On the other hand, as with rape, if the woman does not pursue all avenues, the behavior is likely to persist, although perhaps directed at other women. This may be a heavy burden, but may also be the reason that women consider legal action—it may help other women, whether or not the action is painful to the original complainant.

There is no right answer to when the best action is to pursue legal recourse. Be aware that there are often time limits to when actions can be taken—for example, 180 days for an Equal Employment Opportunity Commission (1-800-669-EEOC) complaint.

## OTHER ACTIONS

Women physicians should also consider their own behavior: Do they discriminate against men? Could their behavior be considered harassment? How do they behave in the office and in leadership contexts?

## SUMMARY

Women physicians should prepare themselves for sexual harassment and sex discrimination because they are common phenomena. Confrontation, often in the form of a simple statement, is and should be the most common method of dealing with unwanted sexually related actions. However, when all else fails, the law is on our side.

## CHAPTER 8

# DISABILITY

ALICIA CONILL AND MARJORIE A. BOWMAN

A disability is an impairment (a physical, mental, or emotional abnormality) that interferes with at least one activity of daily living (bathing, feeding, dressing, or toileting) or independent activity of daily living (balancing a checkbook, paying bills, preparing meals, shopping). Disability of some amount and type is so common as to affect everyone at some time in life. Significant disabilities interfering with major work and life activities are also very common, and their likelihood is underestimated. Approximately one in seven American adults will have a period of disability of 3 months or longer prior to retirement (McNeil 1990). About one in five Americans is estimated to have some level of disability, either mental or physical, with about half of these having a disability that interferes with two or more activities of daily living.

*Disability, at least temporary, is so frequent that a common saying is that those without disabilities are the "temporally abled." It has also been said that being disabled is the one minority group that all of us can join with a split-second notice.*

Like others, women physicians face physical or mental limitations in their abilities that affect their lives. The exact number and type of the disabilities are unknown, but are likely to mirror those of the general population at the same socioeconomic level, with the exception that some may relate specifically to their work. Anecdotal evidence suggests that both physician disability and physician disability insurance rates have increased, but we have no independent verification of this.

## THE COST OF DISABILITY

There are many costs of disability. Disabled individuals may not be able to work. Disabled individuals require medical care, which is expensive both in dollars and time in the United States. Hiring caregivers is expensive, and frequently not covered by insurance. Voluntary caregivers pay a price in terms of emotional well-being and potentially reduced earning capacity. Being less productive and relying on others for basic functions may also be especially emotionally costly for many physicians.

## THE HIDDEN DISABILITIES

When using the word *disability,* many people think of visible problems, such as the inability to walk, paralysis of an arm, or blindness accompanied by physical distortions of the eye. However, most disabilities are not visible, at least not with casual interaction. Many individuals, whose disabilities are hidden, struggle over when and how to make them known.

Hearing loss provides an excellent example. Hearing loss is extremely common and has a significant negative effect. Most hearing loss is not obvious to the casual observer, yet the individual with the hearing loss may have significant impairment in the ability to understand communication. Should the individual say, "I have a hearing loss, please look at me when you speak and speak clearly," or hope they have heard correctly?

Some disabilities or medical problems also create major uncertainty. Breast cancer that is in remission can recur. Multiple sclerosis attacks occur periodically and cause variable levels of disability. Patients with heart disease might have a heart attack. These uncertainties can affect many life decisions and can interfere with interpersonal relationships.

"All physicians have limitations, be they professional (subspecialization is one manifestation), physical, mental, or even attitudinal. The doctor who does not recognize such limitations runs the risk of contracting a severe case of disabling hubris. There are doctors who cannot hear, and those who are deaf to the appeals of their patients. There are doctors who cannot move, and those who are immobilized by prejudice or rigid attitudes. There are doctors who cannot see, and those who are blind to the limits of their own competence. Which of these is the more handicapped?" (Wainapel 1999).

## DISCRIMINATION

Just as with gender or race, disabilities are a source of discrimination, harassment, and belittlement. People are frequently unsure of how to act around a disabled individual and may try to avoid the person by turning away, pretending not to look at them, or avoiding conversation. Thus the disabled person becomes "invisible" (Iezzoni 1996). In the literature, physicians with disabilities bemoan the lack of understanding of their capabilities by licensing boards, their peers, and medical schools (Iezzoni 1996; Rabin et al 1982; Stetten 1981; Wainapel 1999). In a confidential survey of faculty at our medical school (University of Pennsylvania), many of the respondents with disabling conditions reported a strong fear of disclosure. They feared that they would be discounted, that their performance would be negatively reviewed, and that disclosure would not improve accommodation.

## CAREGIVING

Many disabled individuals rely on family or other caregivers for a significant amount of help with daily activities, which makes them feel dependent and the caregiver feel stressed (Andes 1998). In fact, one in four Americans currently provide some kind of care for a person with a chronic condition. More than half of the caregivers say that these responsibilities interfere with their performance and productivity in the workplace. Families and friends are frequently the first to become involved in caring for a disabled person. Women, more commonly then men, find themselves in this role (see Chronic Care in America: A 21st Century Challenge 2001. Robert Wood Johnson Foundation. Princeton, NJ *http://www.chronicnet.org*).

Women physicians may be conflicted between their professional and personal responsibilities. They are driven by their caregiver qualities in both arenas. These stresses are compounded when women physicians find themselves disabled and in the role of the person needing, instead of providing, assistance.

## SOURCES OF INFORMATION

Physicians do not accurately estimate the functional limitations of their patients (Calkins et al 1991). Just as physicians often underestimate the ability of visibly disabled colleagues, or fail to notice them, physicians frequently fail to provide their disabled physician patients with the information that can improve their lives. Information on resources such as low-vision devices, walking aids, and splints or occupational therapy devices, often come from other patients, diagnosis-related support groups, organizations (such as the National Multiple Sclerosis Society), or nonphysician medical personnel (such as occupational or physical therapists). The Internet can be a source of both information and buying opportunities specific to individual needs.

## OTHER MEDICAL CARE

People with disabilities are at risk for not getting preventive care (Iezzoni et al 2000; Nosek and Howland 1997), because of physical, attitudinal, and financial barriers. In spite of the difficulties, routine preventive care such as pelvic examinations and mammograms should be provided.

Similarly, depression is not an expectation or presumption of disability and should be properly diagnosed and treated with medication and therapy. Depression is common with some specific disease states (e.g., multiple sclerosis). Depression is also common in patients adjusting to a chronic disorder and in recently disabled patients.

## AMERICANS WITH DISABILITIES ACT

The ADA (*http://www.eeoc.gov/facts/ada18.html*) has many interesting facets. It protects Americans with *substantial* disabilities from employment discrimination. "Substantial" means a significant limitation or restriction in a major life activity such as hearing, seeing, speaking, walking, breathing, performing manual tasks, caring for oneself, learning, or working. The disability may be real or perceived by the public as real (e.g., a disfiguring injury, past history of cancer now in remission), and the family members and close friends of the disabled are protected against any discrimination on the basis of their loved one's disability. Individuals with prior alcohol or drug dependence are protected.

Legal recourse is available through the Americans with Disabilities Act (1990), but has proved less useful than had been hoped. Complaints must be filed within 180 days. Unfortunately, the percentage of disabled individuals who have returned to substantive work since the passage of the act has been low. The ADA does not apply to employees of small businesses with fewer than 15 employees.

The ADA has been helpful on issues such as accommodation at a job site for an already employed individual who becomes disabled. Patients with disabilities not preventing work have felt empowered to request and obtain special items such as special chairs, telephones, computer accessories, or widened doors for wheelchairs at their current work sites. According to the President's Committee on Employment of People with Disabilities, 80% of job accommodations cost less than $500.

## CONTINUING EMPLOYMENT

Most individuals with a disability are employed in many cases without any special accommodation. For example, the disability may affect the workers' speed, or which ear they listen to the phone with, or their mode of transportation to work, but they are still able to successfully work.

Since passage of the Americans with Disabilities Act, there have been some efforts to assist disabled individuals who have to choose between health insurance (obtained through disability classification) and employment (with associated risks of losing health coverage because their income would exceed financial requirements). These include an executive order in 1998 to facilitate and encourage employment of people with disabilities. This led to the recent passage in both houses of Congress of the Work Incentive Initiative. If this becomes law, this bill would provide for different ways to continue government health insurance (Medicare and Medicaid) when individuals reenter the work force after being disabled.

However, most individuals with *major* disabilities (two out of three) do not work, despite the fact that even with significant and obvious disabilities many individuals can work, particularly with technological aids. Voice-activated dictation systems help those who cannot handwrite or type well, special computer programs can read material to the site-impaired, and improved electric scooters aid in transportation. Some employment issues relate to medical insurance, in that individuals with disabilities may be covered through disability or government programs that they lose if they become employed. The complexities go far beyond medical insurance, and the United States has yet to fully live up to the goal of nondiscrimination against the disabled.

Physicians have additional issues. The long hours, high level of skill, and intensity of work of the typical physician may differently affect physicians with disabilities. But physicians have options that can accommodate their disabilities:

1. Reducing work hours or eliminating night-call
2. Switching to full-time administration, teaching, or research
3. Finding a new location to reduce commuting time or effort

Switching to another specialty may seem appropriate, but it can be difficult to accomplish, as it often requires an additional period of residency training. With the current limitations on residency funding by number of postgraduate years, many programs are reluctant to accept physicians established in another field. However, some switches can be made *within* fields by additional training that does not entail doing a new residency, such as in addiction medicine, disability assessment, or pain management. However, identifying the type of change needed and what position can accommodate a specific disability is not always easy, and trained counselors or occupational therapists may be helpful.

## DISABILITY INSURANCE

Because of the frequency of significant disabilities, disability insurance is highly recommended. Many employers offer disability insurance. However, disability insurance has limitations that must be recognized:

1. Most disability insurance will not cover the first few months of a disability.
2. Some disability insurance only covers individuals if they cannot do *any* job. For a physician to be considered against this standard would be dif-

ficult. Furthermore, physicians need to be insured against their inability to perform within their specific specialty.

3. Most disability insurance does not handle partial disability, or slowly advancing disability, but best provides for the sudden catastrophic event leading to a clear and obvious disability. Because of this feature of disability insurance, much of the cost of disabilities is borne by the individual and the family, not by the insurance company. For example, problems with stamina may limit working hours, but they are not covered by disability insurance. The amount of disability paid to the individual may be based on income at the time the disability occurred, but the individual may have needed to cut back on work hours gradually over the previous several years. Thus, what looked liked good disability insurance turns into little support by the time the individual meets the policy's definition of disability.

4. Disability insurance should include cost of living increases.

All individuals covered by Social Security are also eligible for Social Security disability after two years of disability. However, the rules are strict and possibly applied in a haphazard manner, and there is no certainty that Social Security will cover an individual's disability. Also, the amount of coverage is small.

## FOR WOMEN PHYSICIANS WITH A DISABILITY

- Consult a vocational counselor to assist you with consideration of job accommodations, adaptations, or alternative career directions.

- Consider seeing a mental health therapist. Recognize the phases of adjustment to a new health state. Temporary or not-so-temporary disability is a difficult transition and you should not navigate it alone (even if you are certain you can!).

- Reach out to other women (or men) physicians (locally and nationally) who are facing similar challenges and can serve as sources of support and guidance.

- Contact patient organizations related to the cause of the disability. There are often newsletters, resources, and support groups available.

- If you have questions regarding your legal rights related to employment or insurance, contact an attorney for consultation and advice.

- Consider taking a medical leave to review your options, or request flexibility in work hours or location.

- If you decide to leave your job as it is configured now, although the loss is real, and will be grieved, there will be new possibilities. There will be an opportunity for deeper understanding of patients who entrust their care to you. Our ability to teach our proteges from first-hand knowledge is profound.

- Spunk, desire, and assertiveness are all needed to deal with temporary or permanent disability, and women physicians have proven themselves capable individuals.

"I often refer to my Parkinson disease as my peculiar gift. . . . Please understand me. I do not like my Parkinson disease. It has robbed me of my independence, taken pleasure from my life, stripped away my self-confidence, sapped my energy, depressed my family, separated me from my friends, driven me from my profession, and darkened my future. Yet it has also, as Mark Twain knew, been able to teach me lessons and give me insights that I could have learned in no other way" (Andes 1998).

Being disabled does not take away our essence as an individual, nor is our job our essence. New awareness of disability as an important issue has risen, but is as yet insufficient.

A helpful resource: Schwarz SP. *300 tips for making life with multiple sclerosis easier.* Demos Medical Publishing, New York, New York 1999. The information in this book is also easily applicable to other disabling conditions.

## CHAPTER 9

# PHYSICAL AND MENTAL HEALTH OF WOMEN PHYSICIANS

ERICA FRANK

## PHYSICAL HEALTH

Contrary to myth, there is good evidence that women physicians have healthy personal practices. Health practices are actually better studied in women than men physicians, although the data that exist for men physicians suggest that they also have healthy habits (Wells et al 1984; Wyshak et al 1980). Physician health matters a great deal: not just to the physicians, but because physicians with healthier personal practices are more likely to counsel their patients about prevention issues (Frank, Rothenberg et al 2000).

Regarding total mortality, there are so few older women physicians that there are no good data on women physicians' average ages at death. There are some data (Frank et al 2000) on male physicians' mortality, and the data are encouraging. U.S. men physicians die later (at an average age of 73.0 for whites and 68.7 years for blacks) than do lawyers (72.3 and 62.0 for whites and blacks, respectively), all professionals (70.9 and 65.3), and all white and black men (70.3 and 63.6). Because, as outlined below, women physicians have such good health habits, even when compared to other high socioeconomic status women, it is likely that similarly positive numbers will emerge for them as well.

Much of the data on the physical health of women physicians is from the Women Physicians' Health Study (WPHS, conducted in 1993–1994), which compared a large sample of U.S. women physicians ($n = 4,501$) with an even larger sample taken in 1992 of other U.S. women. This larger sample was the Behavioral Risk Factor Surveillance System (BRFSS) of the Centers for Disease

Control and Prevention and included 1,316 women of high socioeconomic status (SES)—those with graduate or professional degrees and household incomes >$50,000/year—and 35,361 non–high-SES U.S. women. The women physicians generally reported healthy habits, exceeded national health behavior goals in all examined cases, consistently had better health-related behaviors than women in the general population, and even in many cases outperformed other high-SES women. This is especially noteworthy because high-SES individuals usually have healthy behaviors and good health status (Frank et al 1998; Liberatos et al 1988; Winkleby et al 1992), and suggests that women physicians have healthy behaviors beyond those attributable to high income, educational attainment, and occupational prestige. Let's look at these findings in more detail; these and related findings were previously reported extensively (Frank et al 1998).

## Tobacco

Women physicians' most exemplary behavior is abstinence from smoking. For example, compared with women in the general population, women physicians are one-seventh as likely to smoke (only 3.7% smoking in 1994), half as likely to have ever been smokers, and, if they ever smoked, nearly twice as likely to have quit. The great majority (83%) of women physicians who had ever smoked are ex-smokers; a slightly smaller proportion (78%) of high-SES and less than half (47%) of BRFSS women in the general population who have ever smoked are ex-smokers. Of the very few women physicians who still smoke, they average fewer cigarettes per day, and are more likely to have have at least one cigarette-abstinent day in the last year than other women. Another study of executive women (nonphysicians) found a rate of current smoking of 12% (LaRosa 1990).

## Alcohol

Although only one-quarter of women physicians are nondrinkers, the WPHS-BRFSS comparison found that those who drink alcohol report doing so on average only twice a week, averaging fewer drinks per episode of drinking (1.4 drinks) than did high-SES (1.6 drinks) or other women drinkers (2.0 drinks). They also reported almost never drinking large amounts (only 0.1% reported drinking more than four drinks on any one occasion in the past month). The differences between physician and other women's alcohol abstinence rates may reflect physicians' recreational preferences, and/or their scientific assessments of the merits of drinking alcohol, since the contemporary medical literature (Kemm 1993; Stampfer et al 1988) generally supports the healthfulness of low to moderate alcohol consumption along with the harmfulness of high consumption. Most studies of the general population, as well as the one large study of drinking habits of physicians of both genders, have found that women are more likely to abstain from alcohol than are men (Hughes et al 1992).

We acknowledge that, despite the written WPHS survey's confidentiality, women physicians may have felt more compelled than did other women to provide what they perceived to be socially and medically preferred responses. However, WPHS used a confidential, self-administered questionnaire, and BRFSS used a phone interview. This would tend to bias comparisons toward reporting healthier behaviors for the phone-surveyed (nonphysician) population, as they would need to report undesirable behaviors directly to another person. Furthermore, there are few research alternatives to self-reported behavior.

## Diet

According to the same WPHS-BRFSS comparisons, physicians eat somewhat more fruits and vegetables and less fat than did women in the general population but somewhat fewer fruits and vegetables and more fat than other high-SES women. Physicians are more likely to be vegetarians than are other women (8% vs. ≤2%) (White 1999).

## Exercise

Women physicians are also more likely to exercise than are women in the general population (Frank et al, submitted). According to WPHS, only 4% of U.S. women physicians are sedentary, versus 18% of high-SES U.S. women and 31% of all U.S. women. Further, half exercise at least 30 minutes three times a week. However, there is still room for improvement: only 6% exercise with at least moderate intensity for at least 30 minutes five times/week (the American College of Sports Medicine's recommendation for achieving substantial cardiovascular benefit). As in other arenas, there was a strong correlation between personal health habits and likelihood to counsel patients; in a model including confounders, those women physicians who exercised with at least moderate intensity for 30 minutes at least five times/week were half again as likely to counsel patients at every visit to exercise.

## Other Personal Health Practices

Other health-related behaviors also seem to be better among women physicians than among other women. They are half as likely to have a household firearm than are other women (18% of women physicians), and two to six times as likely as others to have tested their households for radon (Baldwin 1998). Finally, they, like other high-SES women, are highly likely to be consistent seatbelt wearers and they are about twice as likely to use postmenopausal hormone replacement therapy (McNagny et al 1997).

## Personal Screening Practices

For all the reported screening and testing parameters that were studied in the WPHS-BRFSS comparison, women physicians outperformed women in the general BRFSS population (with the exception of blood pressure, where they performed equivalently). However, they did not outperform the high-SES women as much. Women physicians outperformed other high-SES women in cholesterol measurements; performed equivalently to them in blood stool testing, procto/sigmoidoscopy rates, clinician breast exam in those aged <40 years, and in mammography; but performed worse in recency of blood pressure measurements, clinician breast exam in those aged 40 years, and Pap smears. It is interesting to speculate about why women physicians with presumably good access to clinical services, although performing well, performed worse than other high-SES women for some screenings. Women physicians may disagree with screening recommendations, such as for Pap smear frequency, particularly if they know they are personally at low risk. They may believe they can adequately perform their own breast exams. Alternatively, however, they may deny their vulnerability, be embarrassed about seeing another health care provider for simple screening services, or have scheduling difficulties.

It is worth noting that the WPHS-BRFSS comparison showed that physicians exceeded year 2000 national goals (as stated in *Healthy People 2000*) for all examined behaviors and screening practices and that neither BRFSS population did so (though the high-SES women met more goals than did the general population of BRFSS women). Given these findings, it is worth considering whether women physicians ought to be deemed a "gold standard" for subsequently establishing national goals. For example, although a 0% smoking rate might be ideal from a health perspective, it is unlikely to be achievable. Therefore, it may be useful to be able to say, "If we took a group of women, gave them every socioeconomic advantage, and placed them in a milieu that discouraged obviously unhealthy behaviors, what smoking rate might one be able to achieve?"

The limited studies addressing the question of the personal health practices of men physicians have also demonstrated a high standard of physicians demonstrating healthy behaviors (Wells et al 1984; Wyshak et al 1980; Frank et al 1998). Compared to the general U.S. male population, men physicians have been shown to more frequently adopt healthy behaviors and to have lower mortality rates; we have data currently showing that they also have lower mortality rates than do male professionals of the same ethnicity (Frank, Biola, Burnett 2000).

## MENTAL HEALTH

How bad can your life possibly be? You've made it professionally, your parents are satisfied, and you can afford to take a trip to the Caribbean when you need a break. And yet there are both real and imagined problems that contribute to some people's impression that women physicians may have compromised mental health.

Although there are significant limitations in the older literature on women physicians' mental health status, broad and emphatically negative statements are often made about women physicians' psychological states. In fact, some of the most persistently cited data about U.S. women physicians concerns their suicide rates. This has helped create some of the toxic myths about what happens to women who are lucky enough to be well educated, well paid, and in a well-respected profession. Some studies examining this subject have found substantially elevated suicide rates for women physicians compared to other categories of women (odds ratios as high as 4 have been reported) (Craig and Pitts 1968; Pitts et al 1979; Roy 1985; Steppacher and Mauser 1974). However, most such studies have been based on very small numbers (between 17 and 49 suicides) (see review in Frank and Dingle 1999). For example, between 1991 and 1993, 48 U.S. physician (and only two female physician) suicides were reported to the American Medical Association (AMA) (Johnston 1996). Further confusing the picture are other problems: suicide rates are probably underreported, death certificates are inaccurate, other methodology issues are also common, and many of the older studies may not be pertinent today.

At the time of the last edition of our book (Bowman and Allen 1990), in our review of suicide rates we concluded that women physicians had a higher rate of suicide than other women but about the same rate as men physicians, whose rate was similar to men in the general public. The same seems true today. The two largest studies (Rich and Pitts 1979; Steppacher and Mauser 1974) on physician suicide were based on AMA data. Steppacher and Mauser (1974) reviewed AMA data on U.S. physician deaths from 1965 to 1970 with confirmation of the cause of death; there were 489 male physician suicides (30.9/100,000) and 41 female suicides (33.6/100,000). The Rich and Pitts (1979) study reviewed deaths from 1967 to 1972 and found a male physician suicide rate of 40.7/100,000 ($n = 544$) and a female physician suicide rate of 39.7/100,000 ($n = 49$). Suicide has historically been thought to account for a third of premature deaths of physicians (Thomas 1976), with an AMA study suggesting suicide was the cause of 3% of male and 6.5% of female U.S. physician deaths (AMA Council on Scientific Affairs 1986). The actual rates (number per 100,000 physicians), as compared to percentage of deaths, are similar for men and women physicians, which are similar to those of white men over 25 years of age (Holmes and Rich 1990; Rose and Roscow 1973), but significantly higher than the suicide rate for white women over 25 years of age. Some studies have noted little if any elevation of suicide rate in U.S. men physicians (odds ratios of <1.0–1.2) compared to other U.S. men (Rose and Roscow 1973; Ullmann et al 1991), but Lindemann et al (1996) concluded from a thorough review of the literature that men physicians' suicide rate was 1.1 to 3.4 times greater than that of the general male population and 1.5 to 3.8 times greater than that of other men professionals. They also concluded that women physicians' suicide rate was higher than that of other women but similar to that of men physicians.

The data on the rate of depression are similarly unclear because of inadequate studies. Several investigations have found that women medical students, residents, and physicians are more depressed than their male counterparts and women in the general population. Suicidal thoughts were reported by 13% of the medical students and 11% of housestaff in a study at a U.S. midwestern medical school (Hendrie et al 1990). A 1987 questionnaire study of 70 British female housestaff physicians found that 46% had scores indicative of depression, with 7% reporting suicidal ideation (Firth-Cozens 1990). These housestaff physicians reported that their most significant stressors were role conflict and sexual harassment; those who were depressed perceived more stress. In

Finland, 22.1% of the male physicians and 25.9% of female physicians reported a history of suicidal ideation and/or attempts (Olkinuora et al 1990). These studies tend to have few numbers and not to be based on rigorous psychiatric diagnoses. However, other investigations have found no difference in the incidence of psychiatric illness between men and women physicians (Watterson 1976) and lower rates of depression in women family physicians than the general female population (Brown 1992). It may be that physicians, including women physicians, have lower rates of suicidal intent but higher rates of completion than women in the general population (Von Brauchitch 1976), perhaps based on a better understanding of suicide methods and likelihood of success. It certainly seems that prior estimates may have substantially exaggerated women physicians' suicide risk.

Information from WPHS is based on a considerably larger and more representative sample than the prior literature, however, and paints a very different and much more encouraging picture. Of course, WPHS surveyed living physicians and cannot provide a suicide rate. But it does provide self-reported depression and suicide-attempt rates. WPHS showed that among women physicians, 19.5% reported having been depressed, numbers comparable to the reported lifetime risk of major depression for all U.S. women (estimated to be between 7–25% by Blazer et al 1994). Similarly, only 1.4% reported having attempted suicide (61 of 4,501 respondents); National Institute of Mental Health (NIMH) data reveal that 4.2% of women in the general population have made a suicide attempt (Moscicki et al 1988).

Various hypotheses have been advanced to explain physician suicide, with suggested contributing factors including psychiatric disorders, substance abuse, alcoholism, stresses of practicing medicine, unrealistic expectations, role conflict, lack of professional support, inadequate psychiatric treatment of physicians, resistance to psychiatric treatment, personality characteristics, and psychosocial factors. Affective disorders, alcoholism, and substance abuse appear to be the most common psychiatric diagnoses among physicians who commit suicide. To a certain extent, WPHS confirmed these hypotheses for women physicians.

According to the WPHS, factors predicting self-reported depression and suicide attempts among women physicians are a history of alcohol abuse or dependence, sexual abuse, or domestic violence; worse current or past physical or mental health; more severe harassment; and a family history of psychiatric disorders. Depression was also more common among those who lived alone, were childless, had a household gun, and had more home stress, and among those reporting working too much, career dissatisfaction, less work control, and more work stress.

Even one death is tragic and essential to try to prevent, and such events require acknowledgment and redress. But it is worth considering that falsely conveying the idea that women physicians may be at elevated risk of suicide might be harmful. It is important for women physicians to know that the trials they go through are normal, many other women physicians have weathered the same problems, they can ask for help, and they can emerge psychologically healthy.

## Vignette: (continued)

ake new forms. It became my "fault" for calling this be-
ver meant to harm me. But, harm me he continued to do.
ional help for the third time and finally made major
ist taught me how the former episodes of abuse became
rent acceptance of abuse, even while I would verbalize a
f the vile behavior. I have learned to carefully recognize
m accepting abnormal levels of guilt for someone else's
aviors are not my fault. I must force myself to take as-
passive or merely verbal actions when the first levels of
cognized. This has gotten easier and easier, and I find it
 some difficult patients!
ds so typical, so typical, of an abused woman. Unfortu-
represent a far greater percentage of women physicians
physicians will admit to themselves or others. My recom-
it now, early, and get help, makes the necessary changes
suming your life.

*Anonymous Woman Physician*

## DOMESTIC VIOl

Histories of domestic
among women physi
general population,
number of other va
Women physicians w
likely to report histor
cigarette smoking. Su
ily where their mothe
stress at home, and
physicians with sexua
depression and suicid
fair or poor reported
bisexual, and to have s
gency medicine.

Overall, women ph
cally. At the same time

## ACKNOWLEDGME

Dr. Arden Dingle help
women physicians and

partially abate and
havior abuse—he ne

I sought profess
headway. My thera
a pattern of transpa
lack of acceptance
early signs that I a
behavior. Their be
sertive rather than
minor abuse are re
even helps me with

I know this sou
nately, I suspect I
than most women
mendation: admit
. . . before it is con

I have been abusec
and be public in ack
anonymous for two r
embarrassment; and le

The episodes of abu
ated my life. As a ch
touched me. I was rap
first and only date, n
drugs, divorced him fo
me. How could I not d

In my abusive marri
I concurrently believed
for his anger over my o
joled, pleaded, talked, a
ior. We talked some mo

## CHAPTER 10

# Ethnicity in Women Physicians

Jada Bussey-Jones and Giselle Corbie-Smith

Other chapters in this book have reviewed many of the challenges faced by women physicians. Although minority women physicians face these same challenges, they may also face the stress of racism: negative racial stereotypes, alienation, racial isolation, and assumptions about intellectual abilities. In addition, practice choices and the academic climate may present unique challenges to minority women physicians. This chapter reviews the personal and professional characteristics of minority women physicians and some of the important issues they face, including racism and ethnically based harassment, affirmative action, and academic promotion.

## PERSONAL CHARACTERISTICS

Most women physicians (75.3%) are self-described as white/non-Hispanic, with 12.6% Asian, 5.1% Hispanic, and 4.2% black. In data from the Women Physicians' Health Study (WPHS) examining racial correlates, half of Hispanics and most Asians were born outside of the United States, whereas nearly all blacks and whites were U.S. born (Corbie-Smith et al 2000). Blacks were less likely to be married, and Asians were more likely to be married and to have children. There were no significant differences among ethnic groups among the average number of children (2.0 for Asian physicians and 2.2 for white, black, and Hispanic). The fathers of Asian and white women physicians had the highest level of educational attainment. This may suggest higher educational debt for Hispanics and blacks after completion of medical school and residency.

## PROFESSIONAL CHARACTERISTICS

According to WPHS data, non-Hispanic white women physicians were more likely to be board certified, whereas Hispanic women physicians were least likely (Corbie-Smith et al 1999). Blacks and Hispanics were more likely to choose primary care specialties and to practice in urban areas. Black physicians are more likely to work in government or "other" settings. Asian physicians earned the most, and Hispanics reported earning the least income. Additionally, ethnic minority women physicians were more likely to report spending time each week on clinical work for which they did not expect compensation.

## WOMEN MINORITIES IN MEDICAL SCHOOL

Minority women are the fastest growing segment of medical school classes. This may be partly because of affirmative action and national initiatives aimed at producing a physician work force that more closely reflects the ethnic composition of the U.S. population (Association of American Medical Colleges [AAMC] 1970, Nickens et al 1994; Petersdorf et al 1990). For example, Project 3000 by 2000, a 1991 AAMC initiative to increase underrepresented minority representation in the physician work force, had seen encouraging initial successes. Although the number of medical school matriculants in general, and minority matriculants in particular, has been declining, minority women have been increasing their representation in medical school at a faster rate than nonminority women and minority men and currently compose about 55% of the minority entering class (Ready and Nickens 1991, Whitcomb 1995).

These advances have been recently jeopardized. The changes in demographic composition of the U.S. population, recent downward trends in matriculation of medical students from groups considered to be underrepresented, and current uncertainty regarding affirmative action bode poorly for ethnic parity in the U.S. physician work force (Hanft & White 1987, Simpson and Aronoff 1998). By 1994 the number of underrepresented minorities in medical school plateaued (AAMC 1998; Nickens et al 1994). In 1997, for the first time since 1988, the number of medical school applicants decreased across all racial and ethnic groups, with the decline sharpest for underrepresented minorities (AAMC 1998). The number of first-year medical students from underrepresented minority groups decreased by 4.0% from 1995 to 1996 and by 7.1% from 1996 to 1997 (AAMC 1998). Given these data, substantial increases in the number of minority medical students would be needed to have the ethnic composition of the United States more closely reflected in the physician work force. It is estimated that by the year 2025, minority groups will compose 37.6% of the U.S. population, with African-Americans and Hispanic-Americans representing 13.0% and 17.6%, respectively (U.S. Census Bureau 1998).

The decline in minority medical students is partly due to anti–affirmative action policies. In fact, in states that implemented anti–affirmative action policies, medical schools witnessed a 12% drop in minority applicants in 1997 and a 22% drop in 1998 (The Pew Health Professions Commission 1998). The term *affirmative action* was first used in the 1960s to describe programs that allowed schools, employers, and other organizations to take race, gender, national origin, or disability into positive consideration in the selection process. Affirmative action was proposed primarily as compensation for previous societal discrimination, as well as a means to provide necessary diversity in the work force.

Before 1968, most minority students were trained at Meharry or Howard medical schools (Wilson and Kaczmarek 1993). The numbers of minority medical students at other medical schools increased, reaching a high of 10% of enrollment in 1974 after a call by the AAMC to medical schools to have student bodies be more representative of the population as a whole (Petersdorf et al 1990). In 1974, Allan Bakke, a white student, filed a successful lawsuit after being denied medical school admission, claiming reverse discrimination. The courts agreed with his complaint (Carlisle et al 1998). Following the Bakke case and others like it, many affirmative action programs were dismantled, and the rate at which underrepresented minority students entered medical school diminished substantially (Carlisle et al 1998; Petersdorf et al 1990).

Those who oppose affirmative action argue that these programs allow less qualified applicants admission into medical school, and thus produce less competent physicians. A study done by Davidson and Lewis (1997) documenting the experience at the University of California–Davis challenges this notion. This study reviewed the Davis affirmative action and other special consideration admissions for 20 years between 1968 and 1987. Data on academic progress, national board examination scores, graduation, residency evaluations, and practice characteristics were reviewed. Regular admission students were more likely to receive an "A" grade or honors, and they had higher scores on parts I and II of the National Board of Medical Examiners examination. However, there was no difference in failure rates of core courses, completion of residency training, or evaluation of performance by residency directors. Additionally, the rates of board certification and practice characteristics were also similar. Although this study will not end the debate on affirmative action, it does show one institution that has had a successful experience with promoting ethnic diversity.

## STRESS, RACISM, AND ETHNICALLY BASED HARASSMENT

Because of smaller numbers and perceived discrimination, minority medical students often feel isolated at predominantly white medical schools. For example, a study by Bonnett and Douglas (1983) of 147 Northeast black medical students revealed that minority medical students believed white students were able to relate better to white faculty and that minority students were more often treated unfairly and were received less enthusiastically by faculty and administration (Bonnett and Douglas 1983). Shervington & Bland (1996) evaluated stress and coping among a small sample of first- and second-year black female medical students and found these students had concerns about issues of racial isolation, negative stereotyping, and negative assumptions about intellectual abilities. Students expressed fear of failure, seeing individual failures not only as personal but as affecting perception of blacks as a whole (Shervington et al 1996).

Other authors have also described personal experiences or observations of ethnically based harassment in medical students and residents. Baldwin and colleagues (1994) reported 23% of all responding second-year residents reported at least one experience of racial or ethnic discrimination during their first year of training. In this cohort, African-American, Asian, and foreign-born residents were more likely to report ethnically based harassment, with prevalences as high as eight times that of white residents. In addition to personal experiences, over 60% of the residents also reported observations of racial or ethnic harassment of colleagues. In another survey of medical students, half of those identifying themselves as nonwhite or Hispanic reported being the target of racial slurs by classmates, faculty, or residents (Sheehan et al 1990).

In fact, perceptions of harassment based on race and ethnicity has been well documented throughout training and clinical practice. Data from WPHS showed that racial minority groups and foreign-born female physicians reported the highest rates of ethnically based harassment (Corbie-Smith et al 1999). Harassment in this study was defined as having "received unwanted physical or verbal attention, propositions, hostilities, or threats." The prevalence of ethnically based harassment in black women physicians ranged from 2 to 10 times the rate in other groups. One-third of black physicians reported harassment before medical school, in school, in training, or in practice. Twenty-five percent of minority women physicians reported harassment in three of these four settings.

In WPHS, harassment prevalences were the same for older and younger physicians, and were not lower among younger minority physicians. The lack of decline may in part be explained by increased awareness of harassment in younger physicians. Alternatively, older minority physicians may have been more likely to train at historically black institutions where harassment experiences might be less common. However, WPHS data also examine harassment experiences after training and raise concerning questions of how increases in the numbers of ethnic minorities may have negatively affected the reception of minorities within the medical field.

There is an emerging literature describing the effect of perceived discrimination or harassment on mental health. Racial discrimination has been shown to be negatively associated with a sense of personal well-being and associated with higher levels of psychological distress (Amaro et al 1987; Jackson et al 1996). In a study of freshmen medical students' perceptions of stress (Murphy et al 1984), 84% of minority students reported stresses related to race. In

WPHS, increasing levels of any type of harassment were associated with more severe work stress in Asian physicians. For all ethnic groups combined, those wishing to change their specialty were more likely to report having been harassed. Although it is not possible to establish causality from these cross-sectional data, this association is of particular concern in light of a 1990 study of young physicians, where white women, black, and Hispanic physicians reported the greatest reservations about and dissatisfaction with medicine as a career (Hadley et al 1992). If career dissatisfaction is caused or worsened by ethnically based harassment, an avoidable condition, these associations should not be taken lightly.

## CAREER SATISFACTION

Satisfaction with the practice of medicine has been suggested as one predictor of the availability of health care providers. Some studies have shown that increasing dissatisfaction with medicine is highest in women and minority physicians, and grows with increasing practice administrative requirements, particularly for younger physicians (Cohen et al 1990; Hadley et al 1992). In addition, physicians who report giving more free or reduced-fee care are most likely to be dissatisfied with medicine (Hadley et al 1992). Ethnic minority physicians are most likely to report providing pro bono clinical services (Corbie-Smith et al 1999). In addition, blacks are most likely to report dissatisfaction with their career, and Hispanic and black physicians are least likely to consider becoming physicians again (Corbie-Smith et al 1999).

## PRIMARY CARE AND UNDERSERVED POPULATIONS

Many studies have shown that physicians belonging to ethnic minority groups play a critical role in reducing disparities in access to care for underserved and minority populations. Patients from ethnic minority populations are more likely to identify their usual source of care as a minority physician's practice and minority physicians report caring for a higher proportion of minority patients (Keith et al 1988; Moy and Bartman 1995). Many surveys have also found minority physicians more likely to choose primary care specialities, and black and Hispanic physicians more likely to practice in nonsuburban areas (e.g., areas more likely to have a physician shortage) (AAMC 1998; Cohen et al 1990; Johnson et al 1989; Keith et al 1985, 1988). In addition, patients cared for in the practices of minority physicians also tend to be sicker and are more likely to be covered only by Medicaid or to be uninsured (Keith et al 1985; Moy and Bartman 1995).

Because minority physicians provide a disproportionate share of the care to sicker and medically indigent patients, they may be most at risk for the financial consequences of inadequate reimbursement, especially in capitated systems, and are particularly dependent on appropriate adjustment and reimbursement for severity of illness. In addition, black physicians also perceive themselves to be more vulnerable to differential treatment by managed care organizations than their white counterparts (Lavizzo-Mourey et al 1996). Because resource consumption is often tracked in strategies to keep costs down, physicians treating a larger number of chronically ill patients may be less attractive to organizations aiming to maximize profits.

## ACADEMIC FACULTY

The modest goal set in 1970 of 12% minority first-year enrollment in medical school has yet to be met. Historically, and currently, a limited pool of minority medical graduates contributes to underrepresentation on medical school faculties. The most recent AAMC data reveal that minority female faculty members account for 6% of all faculty in U.S. medical schools. Of all female faculty in United States medical schools 4.3% are black female physicians, 0.2% Native Americans, 3.6% Hispanics, and 11.5% Asian-Americans (AAMC 2000). Several sources indicate that minority faculty members have lower rank and have slower promotion than their white colleagues (Menges and Exum 1983). Some have suggested that these differences may be partly due to minority faculty being on average younger and more recently entering into academics. However, Palepu et al (1998) examined minority faculty academic rank and controlled for other factors that typically influence promotion: total peer reviewed publications, receipt of research grant funding, proportion of time in clinical activities, gender and tenure status, medical school, department, and years as medical school faculty. These authors found that the differences in rank between minority and white faculty could not be explained by these potential confounders. Although there have been some modest gains in the representation of women among medical school faculties, there has been even less success in increasing the number of minority faculty members.

The factors contributing to these differences in promotion and success in academics based on ethnicity are varied. Economic and financial factors are significant issues for minority students. Black Ph.D. candidates, for example, are more likely to be dependent on their earnings and loans than whites and are less likely to receive federal awards and grants (Levinson and Weiner 1991). Black medical students are also more likely to come from families with lower annual incomes and have higher educational debt compared to nonminority students. Additionally, the overall average debt from medical school cost has increased without proportional increases in faculty salaries (Levinson and Weiner 1991).

Minority faculty members face challenges that parallel those of their colleagues. For example, minorities, like other academic physicians, face the challenge of balancing their time. Previous studies have indicated that minority faculty members believe that they have more requirements for teaching and advising than their colleagues, which becomes a barrier for career advancement (Menges and Exum 1983; Suinn 1982). In addition, because there are fewer minority faculty members, as medical schools strive for diversity in committee memberships many minority female physicians may be at highest risk for increased institutional service obligations (Menges and Exum 1983). Black faculty members are also more likely to report more time spent in student counseling and administrative work and are also more likely to devote more time to patient care and less time to research (Levinson and Weiner 1991; Menges and Exum 1983). These service activities are less likely to result in formal rewards and promotion.

The substantial underrepresentation of minority faculty in medicine results in fewer mentors and role models for students and for junior faculty of color. A study of black students during graduate and professional education found that only one in eight had a true mentor (Blackwell 1982; Levinson and Weiner 1991). Additionally, although white faculty members may serve as mentors, mentors tend to select people of similar racial and gender background as mentees (Blackwell 1982; Levinson and Weiner 1991). Minority women faculty members may be particularly vulnerable to this lack of senior women minority faculty.

## SUMMARY

For minority women physicians, the intersection of gender and race can raise significant challenges throughout training and in practice. Unfortunately, affirmative action policies have had varied successes. Although medical school matriculants now more closely resemble the gender of the U.S. population, racial parity has not been reached. This goal may be difficult to achieve with the disruption of some of the programs that positively considered ethnic minority status in medical school admissions. Additionally, admission to medical school is only the first step toward entering the medical profession. Issues of ethnically based harassment, stress related to racism, lack of mentors, and less professional advancement are a few of the additional challenges that face minority women physicians. In addition to affirmative action initiatives, more programs for mentoring and facilitating the progress of minority medical students and professionals should be encouraged.

## CHAPTER 11

# THE OLDER WOMAN PHYSICIAN

MEREDITH MITCHELL AND ERICA FRANK

As the first generation of physicians that includes substantial numbers of women reaches retirement age, it becomes increasingly important to look closely at this group to see what a feminized future medical work force might look like. How do women physicians who started their careers years ago differ from more recent graduates? What has stayed the same? Answering these questions may help us determine which characteristics are universal among women physicians and which characteristics are age or generation dependent. Examining age-related characteristics may also help us determine how medicine has changed for women and what else may need to be changed. Further, as these women leave the work force, they are leaving openings for younger physicians and setting precedents for when and how women physicians tend to age and retire.

## PERSONAL CHARACTERISTICS

### Family Composition

Data from the Women Physicians' Health Study (WPHS) (Frank et al 1997) show that 63% of the oldest group of women surveyed (age 60–70) vs. 74% of the youngest (30–39) are married (Table 11-1). This is because older women physicians have higher rates of divorce (15% for oldest vs. 7% for youngest) and widowhood (10% for oldest vs. 0% for youngest). Of the oldest women

TABLE 11-1.
PERSONAL CHARACTERISTICS OF WOMEN PHYSICIANS BY AGE

|  | Age | | | | |
|---|---|---|---|---|---|
|  | 30–39 | 40–49 | 50–59 | 60–70 | *p*-value |
| **Relationship status, %** | | | | | |
| Married | 73.9 | 73.1 | 74.1 | 63.4 | NS |
| Separated or divorced | 6.5 | 12 | 13.4 | 15.1 | |
| Widowed | 0 | 1.2 | 2.2 | 10 | |
| Single/never married | 15.1 | 10.1 | 8.9 | 10.8 | |
| Cohabiting | 4.5 | 3.5 | 1.4 | 0.7 | |
| **With children, %** | 61.7 | 76 | 83.7 | 81 | |
| **Average no. of children** | 1.2 | 1.7 | 2.1 | 2.3 | |
| **Mean religiousness score** | 2.2 | 2.2 | 2.3 | 2.2 | |
| **Political self-characterization, %** | | | | | |
| Very conservative | 5 | 5 | 8 | 8 | ≤.0001 |
| Conservative | 22 | 17 | 23 | 24 | |
| Moderate | 36 | 37 | 38 | 36 | |
| Liberal | 29 | 29 | 25 | 24 | |
| Very liberal | 8 | 12 | 6 | 9 | |

physicians, 11% never married compared to 15% of the youngest (although these younger women would seem more likely than the older women to subsequently marry). Similarly, 20% more of the oldest women have children, but the younger women may still be building their families. Overall, the family-related numbers do not seem to have changed much: most women physicians marry and have children.

## Political and Religious Self-Characterization

Religious fervor and the percentage of women physicians who subscribe to different political beliefs also are not very age-dependent. The mean religiousness score [queried in WPHS as "Your religious identity is: very strong (4), strong (3), moderate (2), low (1), none (0)"] is about 2.2 for all age groups of women physicians (Frank et al 1999a). Slightly more (8% vs. 5%; *p* ≤.0001) older than younger women physicians characterize themselves as very conservative politically (Frank 1999). This may suggest either that as physicians age they become more conservative or that women who chose to be physicians 30 to 40 years ago were inherently more conservative. However, there are few other differences or trends in political self-characterization. The largest political group for all ages is moderate (36–38%) (Frank 1999). These data suggest that women with many different beliefs choose to enter medicine, and that this has been the case for at least 40 years.

## Personal Health Habits

Though it has been shown to be untrue (Frank et al 1998a), physicians have been stereotyped as an unhealthy group. The stresses of the profession have been postulated to cause alcohol abuse, smoking, poor diet and exercise habits, and other poor health habits. However, data from WPHS have shown that women physicians, despite busy and stressful lives, have lower rates of smoking and alcohol use and better nutrition and exercise habits as compared to other women in the general population (Frank et al 1998a) (see Chapter 9). Healthy habits have also been found in the few small studies of men physicians that have been conducted. It is interesting to see how women physicians' personal health habits change as they get older. Since older women physicians work less than do younger women physicians (Frank et al 1997), they have more time to devote to other activities, including leisure and health maintenance. This time differential is especially true since the oldest women physicians averaged 0 hours of child care per week vs. 31 hours per week reported by the youngest (Frank and Harvey 2000).

## Smoking

Although few women physicians smoke, even compared with women of similar socioeconomic status in the general public (4% vs. 8%), it is worth noting that women physicians' smoking rates differ by age. Among the oldest group of women physicians, 6% currently smoke as compared to 3% of the youngest group (Table 11-2). These data suggest that smoking rates will continue to decline even more among physicians.

## Exercise

The exercise recommendation for meaningful cardiovascular benefits is at least 30 minutes of exercise at least three times/week (ACSM 1986); 49% of women physicians comply with these recommendations (Frank et al, in revision). Somewhat surprisingly, 55% of older women physicians comply vs. 47% of younger women physicians (Frank et al, in revision). Many people become less

TABLE 11-2.
PERSONAL HEALTH HABITS OF WOMEN PHYSICIANS BY AGE

|  | Age | | | |
|---|---|---|---|---|
|  | 30–39 | 40–49 | 50–59 | 60–70 |
| Current Smoker, % | 2.4 | 3.9 | 6.3 | 6.3 |
| Self-reported sexual abuse, % | 4.6 | 5.2 | 4.5 | 2.0 |
| Has a gun in the home, % | 11.8 | 18.5 | 16.3 | 15.4 |
| Has tested home for radon, % | 18.0 | 17.8 | 17.1 | 11.8 |

active as they get older; however, older women physicians may have more free time, and may become even more aware of the need to stay healthy.

## Depression and Suicide

Depression and suicide attempt rates for women physicians do not seem to be connected with age. Of those ≤45 years of age, 1.6% reported having attempted suicide vs. 1.4% of those >45, and 19.5% of those ≤45 vs. 19.6% of those >45 reported having suffered from depression (Frank and Dingle 1999). Risk of depression for women in the general public has been estimated between 7% and 25% (Blazer et al 1994), so rates for women physicians of all ages do not seem to be elevated.

## Sexual Abuse

Although sexual abuse is reported to occur in about 20% of the general female population (Koss 1988), only 4.7% of WPHS respondents report ever having been sexually abused (Doyle et al 1999). The oldest group of women physicians report histories of sexual abuse at less than half of the rate of the youngest group (2.0% vs. 4.6%; $p$ ≤.001) (Doyle et al 1999). This may be a factor of the changing definition of sexual abuse (i.e., date rape or wife rape) or the more recent emphasis on discussing abuse and healing rather than on hiding the problem for fear of stigmatization. Also most sexual abuse takes place during younger years (Bachman and Saltzman 1995), so older physicians may have tried to forget about or trivialize incidents. On the other hand, these data may signal that sexual abuse among women physicians is in fact becoming more common. If the number of women physicians with histories of sexual abuse continues to grow, the issue warrants further study, because of the possible implications that such abuse may have for a woman and her career. This age-related finding also has interesting potential societal implications: Could it be that we now cope better with psychological and social implications of abuse, allowing victims to remain sufficiently high-functioning that they can become physicians?

## Firearm Ownership

Women physicians are less likely to keep a firearm in their home than is the general public (17% vs. 42%) (Frank and Kellerman 1999). However, older women physicians have a gun in their a home at higher rates than younger women physicians (22% vs 15%; $p$ ≤.05) (Frank and Kellerman 1999). There are several possible reasons for this. The youngest group is much more likely to have young children living in their house and therefore might feel that the risk of having a gun in the house outweighs the possible safety benefits. Older women might be more likely to be living alone due to widowhood or divorce and feel that the gun is necessary for protection. There may also be generational differences in attitudes; it may be more acceptable to older physicians to have a gun because they did not grow up with high rates of gun violence.

## Aspirin and Supplement Use

Both aspirin and supplement use increases with age for women physicians. Among women physicians over 50, 17% report taking at least one aspirin a day vs. 6% among women physicians 50 or younger (Frank, Sperling, 2000). 71% of 65–70 year old women physicians use supplements regularly (≥5 days/week) vs 43% of women physicians age 35–44 (Frank, Bendich, Denniston 2000). Also women physicians with certain diseases take specific supplement at higher rates. Calcium supplements were taken by 76% of those with osteoporosis vs. 25% of those without, and vitamin E was taken by 27% of those with cardiovascular disease (CVD) risk factors such as high blood pressure or high cholesterol vs. 16% of those without (Frank, Bendich, Denniston 2000). These diseases are all more likely to occur in older women.

## Radon Testing

In 1988, the U.S. Environmental Protection Agency recommended that Americans test their homes for radon, a known carcinogen. Estimates of the general population show between 3% and 9% of people radon test their homes (EPA 1992). Women physicians report testing their homes in higher numbers (18%); however, there is a marked difference between the testing frequency of the oldest group of women physicians (12%) and all other age groups (17–18%; $p$ ≤.001) of women physicians (Baldwin et al 1998). This could be because radon has only fairly recently been identified as a health risk, and older women physicians may be less aware of the risks. Alternatively, those with young children may be more concerned about the possible problem than women who live alone or only with a spouse, or those who feel they only have a limited number of years of exposure. Also older women may be less likely to own a home, making testing less of a priority.

## PROFESSIONAL CHARACTERISTICS

## Training, Income, and Practice Setting

Women physicians who completed their training recently (graduates from 1980 to 1989) are more likely to be residency trained and board certified than those who graduated from 1950 to 1960 (Table 11-3) (Frank et al 1997). 98% of recent graduates completed residency training and 64% are board certified compared to 88% and 49% of older graduates (Frank et al 1997). These youngest graduates also have a slightly higher mean income ($102,000 for the younger graduates vs. $100,000/year for the older graduates) (Frank et al 1997). Although the difference is slight, those recent graduates are still building their careers and will likely end up earning more money as they achieve more senior positions. An indication of this is that graduates from 1960 to 1969 earn $123,000/year; these women have probably reached the height of their careers (Frank et al 1997). A possible reason for the difference in salaries is that more recent graduates are more likely to have pursued a higher-paid

TABLE 11-3.
PROFESSIONAL CHARACTERISTICS OF WOMEN PHYSICIANS BY AGE

|  | Age | | | | |
|---|---|---|---|---|---|
|  | 30–39 | 40–49 | 50–59 | 60–70 | *p*-value |
| Residency trained, % | 98 | 94 | 89 | 88 | |
| Board certified in specialty, % | 64 | 72 | 57 | 49 | |
| Mean income in $1000 | 102 | 119 | 123 | 100 | |
| Mean hours of work per week | 49 | 46 | 46 | 42 | |
| Career satisfaction, % | | | | | |
| Always/almost always | 45 | 49 | 54 | 67 | |
| Usually | 37 | 35 | 35 | 25 | |
| Sometimes/rarely/never | 17 | 16 | 11 | 8 | ≤.001 |
| Again become a physician, % | | | | | |
| Definitely/probably | 62 | 70 | 81 | 85 | |
| Maybe/probably or definitely not | 38 | 30 | 19 | 15 | ≤.001 |
| Change specialty, % | | | | | |
| Definitely | 4 | 8 | 8 | 8 | |
| Probably or maybe | 29 | 34 | 36 | 34 | |
| Probably not or definitely not | 67 | 58 | 56 | 58 | ≤.001 |
| Harassment, % | | | | | |
| Gender-based | 48 | 49 | 47 | 40 | ≤.01 |
| Sexual | 40 | 38 | 27 | 24 | ≤.001 |
| Ethnic harassment, % | | | | | |
| Total | 12 | 14 | 13 | 11 | |
| Hispanic | 9 | 33 | 18 | 14 | ≤.05 |
| Black | 60 | 70 | 52 | 71 | |
| Other | 42 | 31 | 32 | 47 | |
| Asian | 35 | 34 | 25 | 26 | |
| White | 6 | 6 | 7 | 6 | |

specialty compared to older graduates, many of whom became primary care physicians. More of the oldest graduates have a solo or government practice than the youngest, who primarily are in group or hospital practices. This could be an indication of how factors like managed care are changing health care. It should also be noted that recent graduates work an average of 49 hours per week, whereas the older graduates average 42 hours per week (Frank et al 1997).

## Career Satisfaction

An important issue to look at with older physicians is career satisfaction. Data from WPHS (Frank et al 1999b) show that the among the oldest group surveyed (60 to 70 year olds), 67% of women physicians are always or almost always satisfied with their careers vs. 45% of the youngest group (30 to 39 years

---

### Vignette

My father, who is now 92 years young, played a key role in my becoming a physician and for any success I've had in the profession of medicine.

I've wanted to be a doctor since I was 4 years old. To that end, I asked Santa Claus for a doctor's kit that year and for the next 3 years. However, for reasons I couldn't figure out, a nurse's kit kept appearing under the tree every Christmas morning for 4 consecutive years. By age 7 I decided to rebel silently (certainly not in character), and didn't open the kit.

After 2 days, my Dad asked me what was wrong with the doctor's kit, and I told him that what I had was a nurse's, not a doctor's, kit. He looked puzzled and asked me what the difference was. I showed him the white nurse's cap with the big red cross on it and said, "Doctors don't wear caps; they wear white coats." He told me that he'd fix that right away and left the room. He returned in a few minutes with a scissors and an old white shirt. He then cut out the red cross and taped (a guy thing; my Mother later sewed) it on to the rolled up sleeve of his old shirt. I put it on and I knew that I would become a doctor, no matter what happened.

The other major thing he did that secured my success in medicine was that he taught me how to play poker. Except for developing a memory for what had been played, the cards were incidental. He taught me how to observe people's reactions in order to determine what they might be thinking. I now play poker every day in my work but never with cards.

Thank you, Poppie, which is his current title according to his seven great-grandchildren.

*Dr. Catherine DeAngelis*

---

old) ($p \leq .001$). In addition 85% of the oldest vs. 62% of the youngest women physicians ($p \leq .001$) would definitely or probably again be doctors if given the choice.

These statistics may sound surprising, considering that many conditions for women physicians have supposedly only gotten better over the past 40 years; shouldn't younger physicians be happier with their careers? However, older women are much further removed from the long hours and erratic schedules associated with training and early establishment of practices, and may be more immune to or removed from the negative aspects of current practice environment. Also as physicians approach retirement age they are more likely to work fewer hours (Chan et al 1998; Frank et al 1997), or they may be more able to only do work that they enjoy instead of trying to build a practice or gain tenure. Young women physicians may be more likely to feel significant stress because they are simultaneously trying to build careers and raise young children. Another reason is that older women physicians may feel "pioneer pride"; they are especially happy with their position because they accomplished something that few of their contemporaries were able to do. The youngest women physicians were also five times more likely to have student loan debts to repay than the oldest women physicians; they were also 91 times more likely to have large debts ($25,000 to >$100,000) (Frank and Feinglass 1999). Anxiety about repaying loans may affect career satisfaction.

Older women physicians were modestly more likely to want to change their specialties (8% vs. 4% for the youngest women physicians). This makes sense, despite higher career satisfaction for older physicians, because older women physicians may have had more limited specialty choices when they went through training; 73% of the oldest women physicians are in primary care as opposed to 66% of the youngest group ($p \leq .002$). Also the youngest women physicians may have more enthusiasm for their specialty because it is a more recent choice, and they may not yet have had time to tire of their job or routines, or to change their interests or priorities.

The differences between older and younger physicians in career satisfaction, desire to again be a physician, and desire to change specialty may be due to the previously suggested practical reasons, in which case the next 30 years should show the same trend: today's recent graduates will report more career satisfaction as they age. However, it could also show a difference in attitudes or expectation among the generations, which would mean that younger women physicians might inherently be less satisfied with their positions, possibly because of recent changes in medicine such as managed care or because of higher expectations. These possibilities merit further tracking and research, to help prevent women from leaving medicine or being unhappy in their profession.

## Counseling

Although a Canadian study shows that younger physicians are more likely to follow recommendations in prevention and health promotion (Robb 1997), WPHS data show that women physicians under and over 50 have nearly the same frequency of counseling patients on 14 counseling and screening items (Frank et al 2000). Much stronger predictors of counseling were whether the physician was in primary care and whether the physician personally practiced the specific healthy behavior.

## Harassment

### Sexual and Gender-Based Harassment

Harassment is another aspect of the careers of women physicians that seems as though it should have only gotten better over the past 40 years. Gender-based and sexual harassment have received so much public attention in recent times that it seems like women should be experiencing less and less of it. However, WPHS data (Frank et al 1998b) suggests that this is not the trend for women physicians.

In WPHS, 48% of the youngest group (30–39) reported ever experiencing gender-based harassment in a medical setting, as opposed to 40% of the oldest group (60–70; $p \leq .01$). Sexual harassment figures are even further apart for the two age groups (40% for the youngest vs. 24% for the oldest; $p \leq .001$). These data seem surprising because our society has supposedly become much more enlightened on the issue of sexual harassment. However, this enlightenment may actually cause the difference. WPHS data are self-reported, and women may differ in their ideas of what type or severity of activity constitutes harassment. The older population of women probably has a different definition from the generation that was exposed to women's liberation and the Clarence Thomas–Anita Hill hearings at an earlier age.

Women today may be more comfortable labeling inappropriate behavior as harassment. Also harassment seems to be most acute during training, and older women physicians are further removed from their training and may have forgotten or trivialized incidents that occurred decades before. Despite possible differences in the reporting of harassment by older and younger women physicians, the idea that sexual harassment is committed only by older, sexist physicians and will vanish as such physicians retire seems to be inaccurate. Perceptions of sexual harassment remain high for younger physicians—possibly even higher than that of their predecessors. It is very important to be aware that sexual harassment is still a problem because it has been associated with depression and higher career dissatisfaction in female physicians and others.

## Ethnicity-Based Harassment

Ethnicity-based harassment also remains a problem for women physicians. Here, however, the numbers for different age groups are not significantly different. The rates remain high, signifying that ethnicity harassment has been and remains a problem (see table 11-3) (Corbie-Smith et al 1999). Of particular note is that 71% of oldest vs. 60% of youngest black physicians report ethnicity harassment (though the difference not statistically significant) (Corbie-Smith et al 1999). This is very high compared to 6% of both the youngest and oldest white women physicians having experienced ethnicity harassment.

The fact that these numbers have changed minimally is cause for concern. Although younger women may report harassment in higher numbers because of increased sensitivity, older women physicians may actually have experienced less harassment because they were more likely to have trained in historically black schools where ethnic harassment might not be as severe. It seems that ethnicity harassment is something that both older and younger women physicians of color have frequently experienced.

## RETIREMENT

Many physicians may feel that the standard retirement age of 65 is too young for them (Robb 1997). In a profession where so much time and effort is put into training and career satisfaction is so high, a 35-year career may simply not be long enough. This may be particularly true for women physicians as they likely will have longer life expectancies (given their healthy personal practices and other social/biological advantages) than do their male counterparts.

There are age-related practice differences. For example, as physicians age they do fewer surgeries, less trauma work, and fewer deliveries and obstetric procedures (Robb 1997). They also see fewer younger patients but more older and rural patients.

So how to best utilize this large and growing resource? One retired physician suggests that retired doctors be recruited to give advice and supervision to elderly patients (Hall 2000), since they have shared and are continuing to share similar experiences. This suggestion may also help relieve physician's fear losing their "doctor identity" (DeFries 1998). After having been identified and also identifying themselves as physicians for so many years, the prospect of losing that identity may be frightening or frustrating for many.

## CHAPTER 12

# WOMEN IN MEDICAL SCHOOLS AND ACADEMIA

MARJORIE A. BOWMAN

As noted in Chapter 1, women did not officially enter medical schools in the United States until the latter half of the 1800s. Women have now become nearly half of the medical students, and a substantial minority of faculty. The number of women in major leadership positions in medical schools has expanded dramatically but remains quite small.

The number of women entering medical school rose dramatically in the 1970s and 1980s from 9.4% in 1969–70 to 28% in 1979–80, to 38% in 1989–1990, then rose more slowly to 43% in 1997–98. (Bickel et al 1998). Women made up the majority of new medical students at 20 U.S. medical schools for 1997–98 (Bickel et al 1998). Women comprised 36% of residents in 1997–98.

As the acceptance rate into medical school for women has not varied much from that of men for most of this century (Bickel et al 1998; Johnson 1983), part of the reason for lower numbers for women must be lower application rates. If women were accepted at the same rate as men, why were not more applying?

## CAREER PRESELECTION

The process by which women are culled out begins early in life. Sex-role socialization begins at birth (Crovitz 1980). Women, in general, have lower evaluations of their abilities than men (Crovitz 1980, Fiorentine 1987). Many women who could be classified as potential physicians on the basis of high school grades and abilities do not even go on to college (unpublished data, Sandra K. Wilson, American Institutes for Research, Palo Alto, California). This is partially confirmed by the higher percentage of women admitted directly from high school to a special combined undergraduate/medical school program (Herman and Veloski 1981). There is an equal ratio of men and women who enter college premedical programs (Fioretine 1987), but women with moderate and low levels of academic performance in college are significantly less likely than men with similar levels of academic performance to apply to medical school. Women medical students indicate that their parents were less supportive of their decision to study medicine than is reported by men (Bickel et al 1998). Thus, many possible future physicians are turned away early or did not persist with their career aspirations. A societal influence has placed certain values and expectations on the role and abilities of women, which women, in turn, have internalized.

---

*In* See Jane Win *(Rimm S, Three Rivers Press, 2000), Dr. Rimm reports on the results of over 1,200 women who were happy and successful at work and at home. The common childhood experiences of these successful women were that parents had high expectations of them; they learned to compete; they were involved in significant activities (such as Girl Scouts, sports, music, and other hobbies); and their mothers or other women close to them were strong role models.*

---

Subtle discrimination by medical schools could also be a factor. The fact that women were admitted in greater numbers during the World War II years when men were less available, and admitted in lower numbers again afterward, could suggest discrimination.

As late as 1970, the Women's Equity Action League filed suit against all medical schools, charging that they were discriminating against women, leading to low numbers of women in medical school.

Women may need to be more committed than men to get into medical school (Matthews 1970). Women candidates may hear about the perceived lack of hospitality of medical schools and decide not to apply; i.e., a subtle feedback loop to the applicant pool exists. Even in recent years, women students interviewing for medical school are more likely to be asked questions about their plans for marriage and family (one-third of the time) compared to men (one-tenth of the time); men were more likely to be asked what influenced their decision to enter medicine and their specialty plans (Marquart et al 1990). Whether or not subtle discrimination could be proven, certainly the number of women applicants and students increased dramatically in the last half of the twentieth century.

## MINOR DIFFERENCES IN ACADEMIC PERFORMANCE

Men tend to do slightly better in the sciences and basic science years of medical school, and women do slightly better in the nonscience classes and clinical years. This has been consistent for 20 years (Case et al 1993). On the MCAT (Medical College Admission Test), men perform better in physics, quantitative, chemistry, and biology, but women had higher nonscience grade point averages in college (Case et al 1993). Scores on Part I of the National Boards of Medical Examiners (NBME) test (taken after the basic science portion of medical school) were significantly different for women and men; women had a mean score of 455 and men a score of 492 (Dawson et al 1994). Differences persisted when MCAT scores, undergraduate grade point averages, and other prematriculation measures were considered (Dawson et al 1994). Case et al (1993), after controlling for the prematriculation differences, found the gender differences in scores on part I and II were reduced for the areas in which men had higher values on the prematriculation measures (for example, quantitative scores and physiology score), but the magnitude increased for the areas in which the differences favored women (for example, behavioral sciences and psychiatry on part II). With the introduction of the United States Medical Licensing Examination (USMLE) by the NBME and Federation of State Medical Boards in 1992, the same gender question has been reconsidered (Case et al 1996). Once again, women received slightly lower passing rates on step I (similar to part I) on the first try but had indistinguishable ultimate passing rates. On step II, the percent passing was equivalent for men and women. In another study (Huff and Fang 1999), at higher MCAT scores men were more likely than women to experience academic difficulty. The only information from board examinations once the physicians are out in practice is from the American Board of Internal Medicine examination, which finds women overall performing less well than men, but with major gains in performance of the women from 1973 to 1982 (Norcini et al 1985); interestingly, middle-aged women outperformed middle-aged men.

---

*Women and men's brains function differently: girls speak sooner and read faster; women's brains respond more intensely to emotion; women's neuronal activity is more greatly distributed throughout the brain for all activities; women's memories outperform men's; and women's brains age more slowly (Hales D. If you think we think alike, think again.* Reader's Digest, *April 1999: 108–112).*

---

Women outperform men in areas related to women's health. In the University of Arizona's Objective Structured Clinical Examinations (Rutala et al

1991), female students scored higher than the men where there was a female standardized patient. Female students traditionally score better in NBME part II in obstetrics and gynecology and pediatrics (Case et al 1993). In the USMLE step II, written patient-vignette cases were varied by sex of the patient (Case et al 1999). The female students overall performed slightly better, but most significantly better on traditionally female disorders.

Noncognitive rather than cognitive factors appear to be more important predictors of medical school achievement for women than men students (Calkins et al 1987; Oggins et al 1988; Willougby et al 1979). Oggins et al (1988) hypothesized that women should do better if a situation demands person-related tasks (such as in clinical clerkships) because of women's higher "communal" orientation, i.e., motivation by social values, including helping, affiliation with others, and social involvement. Her data supported this presumption and found that written evaluations of men's clerkships were better predicted by prior academic achievement and women's by their communal orientation. This was in spite of the fact that the women did not have statistically significant higher ratings for person-oriented values with the exception of "work with people." However, she did not find that women's clinical grades were more related to social skills than men's, a fear that many women have. Solomon et al (1993) also found no gender bias in preceptors' ratings of third-year medical students.

There is little information on performance in residencies. Gender-related clinical evaluations have been found in internal medicine residencies. In one internal medicine residency, male attending physicians give male residents slightly higher scores than female attending physicians did; women residents were rated similarly by both (Rand et al 1998). In another, women were rated higher than men on humanistic qualities, and men were rated higher on procedures and medical knowledge (Day et al 1989).

Attrition rates from medical school of both men and women are low and quite similar (Braslow and Heins 1981; Huff and Fang 1999). After 4 years in medical school, 96% of men and 95% of the women still are in school (Huff and Fang 1999). There is also little information on attrition from residency. In one study of attrition from surgical residencies (1993 entering cohort), women and men from U.S. or Canadian allopathic medical schools had the same attrition rate (9%); residents who were minorities or from international medical schools had higher attrition rates (Kwakwa and Jonasson 1999). Other studies of attrition from residency are older, and their current pertinence is unclear.

Overall, the differences between men and women in academic achievement are minimal and are unlikely to determine long-term success or skill as a practicing physician.

## WOMEN AND MEN EXPERIENCE MEDICAL SCHOOL DIFFERENTLY

Women report fewer role models (Bright et al 1998) and much more sexual harassment and general harassment during medical school and residencies (see

Chapter 7). Both the lack of role models and the perception of harassment by current students may discourage other women from applying to medical school. Women are also much more likely to report being mistaken for a non-physician than are men (92% vs. 3%, $p <.0001$) and feel their medical school experience is significantly affected by their gender (60% vs. 25%, $p <.001$) (Bright et al 1998). Women are more likely to feel they must overcome a fear of failure (31% vs. 19%, $p <.01$) (Bright et al 1998).

## WOMEN AND MEN HAVE DIFFERENT EXPERIENCES DURING TRAINING

Women medical students may see fewer male patients than do men medical students (Wollstadt et al 1990), particularly for sexually related examinations. Anatomy and physical diagnosis text illustrations are more likely to be of men than women (Mendelsohn et al 1994), reinforcing the idea of the normal person as a 70-kilogram man.

## WHY DO WOMEN PHYSICIANS CLIMB THE ACADEMIC LADDER SLOWLY?

Women represent 26% of 1998 medical school faculty (Bickel et al 1998) compared to 24% of all physicians in the United States in 1997 (American Medical Association data). However, women are only 22% of associate professors and 11% of professors (Bickel et al 1998), and the prevalence of tenure for women is 17% compared to men's 37% (Bickel et al 1998). Another recent study (Nonnemaker 2000), using data from the Association of American Medical Colleges, found that there were about 10% more women on the faculty than would be expected. Nonnemaker (2000) found that the distribution of women across ranks had not changed much in two decades. In this study about 34% of men faculty and 12% of women faculty became full professors; unexplained disparities existed in basically every specialty.

What do we know about the reasons for the disparities between men and women physicians in terms of rank and tenure? The first, and certainly a major, reason is age: women physicians are, on average, younger than men physicians, and thus have not had the opportunity to reach the usual career length for higher ranks. For example, an in-depth study at the Columbia University College of Physicians and Surgeons found similar rates of promotion when time in rank was considered (Nickerson et al 1990).

However, the data available are not consistent. Carr et al (1993, data from 1986) found a problem for women faculty in general internal medicine, cardiology, and rheumatology combined: women were promoted less frequently then men when 10 variables were considered (Carr et al 1993), whereas the same authors found no differences in the same survey data when considered for general internal medicine alone (Carr et al 1992). A nationwide sample

## Vignette: The Lonely Road Less Traveled

My favorite poem growing up was "The Road Less Traveled" by Robert Frost. It seemed appropriate that I found myself training in urology in the early 1980s—the only woman in the residency program. Since then, I have spent a great deal of time trying to come to grips with my years of professional isolation and attempt to make sense out of the endless number of "misunderstandings" with male peers and faculty. The feelings of depression and inadequacy were never ending, punctuated by emotional outbursts that didn't make sense even to me. Upon reflection, I formulated my "Ding to Dent" theory.

During training, I was constantly bombarded with inappropriate remarks and subtle inequities that I didn't have the time or energy to acknowledge. Superficially, I would tell myself, "No big deal." Each of these little events was a "ding" to my self-esteem. After enough "dings," a dent appeared, triggered by just another seemingly "No big deal" remark or action. When the "dent" occurred, there was no suppressing emotion—for me, anger or tears. The perpetrator of the most recent "ding" would always be totally mystified by my inappropriate response to "nothing."

I have learned to deflect or process the "dings" as they occur. I stopped second guessing myself as to whether I was being too sensitive. Most important, I have realized the importance of finding a work supportive environment. Trailblazing is a part of what I do, but I have learned to stop along the way at friendly villages.

*Tamara G. Bavendam*

survey in 1991 found that, after 11 years on the faculty, men were more likely to have been promoted than women (Tesch et al 1995).

One of the best studies on this issue highlights the multiple factors that influence the promotion of women faculty was a 1995 nationwide survey of a stratified random sample of full-time salaried faculty Carr et al (1998). In Carr's study, the following factors could be the women's decisions or at least somewhat under their own control:

- Women worked fewer hours per week. These differences were not adjusted for specialty, a major covariate of hours worked (surgeons typically work longer hours, but fewer women are surgeons). The difference in work hours was limited to women with children (54 hours per week), whose hours were about 9% lower than women without children. Women without children and men with or without children all averaged about 59 hours a week.

- Women faculty were less interested in the leadership role of department chair, whether or not they had children (although differences were more marked between men and women with children than those without children).
- Women had more responsibility for child care, spent more time doing it (for those with children, 22 hours per week compared to men's 14 hours), and were more likely to have responsibilities for other nonchild dependents.
- Women faculty reported more limitations on travel and weekend work because of child care responsibilities.

The following factors could be considered institutional factors:

- Women faculty were less likely to receive research money from the institution (47% vs. 57%).
- Women faculty had about 20% less secretarial support.

These two effects were limited to the women faculty with children which suggests this was not discrimination strictly on the basis of gender.

Overall, Carr et al (1998) found that the women faculty had a similar division of time spent for research, teaching, patient care and administration, and a similar level of research grants, but had many fewer publications (23 compared to 36, unadjusted); the difference in publications was limited to women faculty with children compared to men faculty with children. The rate of publication alone is sufficient to account for much slower rates of promotion. Many publications are written nights and weekends, rather than during the workday. The extra hours women faculty who have children spend on child care could easily translate into the differences in the number of publications (Table 12-1).

However, looking at the adjusted numbers, one could have another interpretation: men faculty with children (who tend to have spouses who take care of household responsibilities) publish more than the other three groups, all of

TABLE 12-1.
PUBLICATIONS IN ACADEMIC GENERAL INTERNAL MEDICINE BY GENDER
AND PARENTING STATES

|  | Average Number of Publications (Adjusted) |
| --- | --- |
| Women Faculty with Children | 18.3 |
| Women Faculty without Children | 17.6 |
| Men Faculty with Children | 29.3 |
| Men Faculty without Children | 20.5 |

These means were adjusted for medical school, race, year of first faculty appointment, age, and marital status.
Source: Adapted from Carr et al 1998 with permission.

whom are likely to have substantial household responsibilities, even if it is just for themselves as single individuals.

Another, earlier, nationwide survey (Tesch et al 1995) found no relationship of promotion to the number of children but found a similar 10% lower work hours (53 vs. 58 hours) and fewer publications by women. Even when these productivity factors were taken into account, though, women were less likely to have been promoted. Importantly, the attrition rate from academic medicine was found in this study to be similar for women and men. The women had similar rates of any grant support but were less likely to have National Institutes of Health (NIH) grants, had more time in patient care, were more likely to be in primary care, and had less protected time for research.

## MENTORS

Mentors are important (Levinson et al 1991), although they were not explicitly considered by Carr et al (1998). Physicians who have mentors publish more (Bland and Schmitz 1986). Women seem to feel less supported, have less mentoring, and feel less confident in their academic roles (Carr et al 1992, 1993, 1998). As recently as 1988, 67% of full-time faculty women under the age of 50 reported no current professional relationship with a successful role model (Levinson et al 1989). Certainly, the lack of women in higher leadership at schools means women faculty have few same-sex high-ranking role models.

---

*Kling (Psychological Bulletin 1999; 125:470–500) analyzed data from over 200 studies and found that there were only minor differences in self-esteem between males and females, including at adolescence, when there was a temporary, slightly increased gap.*

---

Dr. Bernadine Healy (1992), formerly the director of the NIH, noted that women and men had similar success rates with NIH grants, although women requested less money. This was because much of the women's money came from the First Awards (R29s) for new investigators; in 1990, women held 18% of dollars for competing traditional research projects and 28% of First Awards (R29's) (Pinn 1992). As the First Awards can lead to additional awards, this may mean more women will be getting more NIH competing traditional awards in the future.

Benz et al (1998) reviewed the literature and concluded that there was evidence of discrimination against women faculty, less support for research activities and career development, lack of effective mentoring relationships, structural inflexibilities (such as little support for part-time status), isolation among women who achieve promotion, and selection bias. Women also are more modest and less likely to see themselves qualified for top positions even when their credentials are similar (Eagly et al 1995).

## ARE WOMEN PHYSICIANS BREAKING THE GLASS CEILING?

No, but there may be slight bends or cracks. Just as in other areas of physician leadership, women are underrepresented at the top in medical schools. The average medical school has one woman department chair (range 0–5); 34 schools have no women department chairs, with two admitting that they have *neither any* women division directors *nor any* women department chairs (Bickel et al 1998, data for 1997–98). Nine medical schools out of 125 had women deans in 1997–98.

## WHAT CAN BE DONE TO INCREASE WOMEN PHYSICIANS' ADVANCEMENT?

Major groups, such as the American College of Physicians (see Sidebar) and the Association of American Medical Colleges (AAMC Project Committee 1996), and individual organizations (Heid et al 1999) or medical school departments (Benz et al 1998), have proposed solutions. In general, the most important factor for achievement is to make increasing women physicians'

What Should be Done?

The American College of Physicians (ACP) reviewed the literature on women and minority physicians on medical school faculties and recommended the following (ACP 1991):

Position 1: The ACP recommends that academic institutions reaffirm their commitment to increase the numbers of qualified women and minority physicians on their faculties.

Position 2: The ACP urges all medical schools to adopt institutional strategies that will foster the promotion of minorities and women from junior to senior faculty positions:

1. Wide dissemination of written guidelines for tenure and promotion procedures.

2. Establishment of a formal career counseling program for junior faculty.

3. Establishment of a faculty development program.

4. Development of flexibility in tenure and promotion procedures that allow faculty to accommodate personal and family responsibilities while continuing academic work.

5. Encouragement of the involvement of women and minorities on policy-making and faculty recruitment committees.

6. Establishment of a formal monitoring process.

advancement a true goal. Multiple factors have led to our current circumstances, and repeated efforts at multiple levels will be required to make a difference. Women physicians, their partners, employers, coworkers, employees, the government, and institutions are all a part of changing our current milieu and attitudes.

## WHAT CAN A WOMAN ACADEMIC PHYSICIAN DO?

Advancement of a woman's academic career is not just the responsibility of the institution. There is much personal responsibility the woman physician can take:

1. Have professional short- and long-term goals so that you can design your path accordingly. Write them down. Regularly review them, at least annually.
2. Choose your job well, one that fits you and your long-term desires.
3. Know rank and tenure systems, particularly that of your institution, both what is written in the policy manual and what is not written but important.
4. Seek out mentors early; nurture the relationships, and ask questions, seek advice, and suggest ways mentors can help you. For example, ask them to suggest what committees you should be on; ask them to submit your name as a possible speaker for a meeting, or as a coauthor, or as a co-investigator, or as a committee member. Ask for honest feedback. Mentors do not all need to be at your home institution. Remember, mentors are often honored that you see them as expert.
5. Network inside and outside the institution. It will be easier to find someone to help with a portion of the grant, to write your letters for promotion, or to have someone invite you for a visiting professorship if you already know them and they know you.
6. Mentor others. You learn from doing.
7. Find other individuals with similar rank to discuss how they are managing. Share specific information, such as salaries.
8. Attend seminars designed for women, or about managing career/family, or about rank and tenure systems.
9. Once or twice a year, meet with your supervisor (such as division director or department chair) to review progress, set goals, and get evaluation of your past performance. Know your strengths and admit your weaknesses. Show how you will overcome your weaknesses.
10. Seek out pertinent additional training often.
11. Be assertive, but not negatively aggressive. Good interpersonal skills are important to long-term success.
12. Maintain a realistic perspective about how you are doing professionally compared to other physicians at your experience level.

## SUMMARY

As more women have entered medical school, some women's issues have ameliorated, but there are a few important issues that have yet to disappear. Increasing numbers and percentages of women will advance the academic ladders, and other, more junior, women will have expanded mentors and role models. The picture is increasingly rosy, and we look forward to the changing face of medicine.

## CHAPTER 13

# WOMEN PHYSICIANS IN PRACTICE

MARJORIE A. BOWMAN AND ERICA FRANK

Women and men physicians show substantial differences in their professional practices, primarily in types of specialties, traditional productivity measures (women's are lower), and income (women have less). However, income per hour is about the same when multiple factors are considered, and satisfaction with careers is both high and similar for women and men physicians.

## SPECIALTY

One of the striking differences between men and women physicians is which specialties they choose. In fact, gender is the strongest factor in specialty choice by physicians. Although women's specialty choices have become slightly more like those of men over the years as more women entered medicine (e.g., moving into surgical specialties more), the choices remain remarkably different. Table 13-1 highlights these differences. The largest differences are in pediatrics, psychiatry, and obstetrics and gynecology, where women are overrepresented, and in surgery, where women are underrepresented. These same fields were chosen by higher or lower percentages of men and women in 1953 (Dykman and Stalnaker 1957).

Why are there specialty choice differences by gender? Overall, in medicine, the reasons for choices of specialty have remained about the same from the 1930s to 1990s: intellectual content of the specialty, challenging diagnostic problems, interest in helping people, opportunity to make differences in people's

TABLE 13-1.
SPECIALTY CHOICE OF WOMEN VS. MEN PHYSICIANS

| Specialty | Women Physicians (%) (WPHS, 1993) | Women Physicians (%) (AMA, 1997) | Men Physicians (%) (AMA, 1997) |
|---|---|---|---|
| Pediatrics | 16.4 | 17.4 | 5.7 |
| Internal medicine | 21.2 | 22.2 | 24.0 |
| General/family practice | 12.0 | 14.2 | 14.7 |
| Psychiatry | 11.3 | 9.5 | 6.0 |
| Obstetrics/gynecology | 8.2 | 8.4 | 5.6 |
| Anesthesiology | 5.6 | 5.2 | 5.7 |
| Surgery | 6.5 | 5.4 | 20.8 |
| Radiology | 3.3 | 4.3 | 5.5 |
| Pathology | 3.6 | 3.3 | 2.3 |
| Other | 11.9 | 10.1 | 9.8 |

Source: Adapted from Frank et al 1997; Gonzalez ML, AMA data at http://www
.ama-assn.org/advocacy/healthpolicy/x-ama/gender.htm, with permission.

lives, and consistency with personality and belief that one had the required skill
or ability (Krol et al 1998). These aspects of specialty choice are important to
both women and men.

Pediatrics and obstetrics-gynecology are related to mothering and childbearing, which are very important for women in our society, and may be why
these specialties seem consistent with the personality of women. As we review
in Chapter 14, women are less likely to be oriented to procedures, consistent
with their lower selection of surgery. Some may speculate that the specialty se-
lections result from a desire for specific types of work hours or work settings,
but this is difficult to justify, as the on-call responsibilities may be heavy for
both pediatrics and obstetrics-gynecology.

There are other theories on the differences in specialty selection by gender.
The perceived femininity of the specialty may be a factor, but there is little literature support for this. In one study (Beil et al 1980), only in the field of pediatrics, which was perceived as feminine, was there a greater proportion of
women and men with higher femininity scores. Women may also be steered toward (Ducker 1978) and desire less prestigious specialties, as their specialty
choices are on average less prestigious. The compatibility with future families
is a draw. Women surgeons are less likely to be married. Is this their choice?
The result of work hours? The result of their appeal to men as a spouse? In one
study (Burnley and Burkett 1986), women medical students considering surgery were more likely to agree that physicians need to sacrifice their personal
lives for their work.

The higher percentage of women among international medical graduates
also influences national statistics. International medical graduates differ from
U.S. graduates in their specialty choices. The specialties of international medi-

## Vignette

When I was a child—to be honest, well into my teen years!—I wished I were a boy. Boys had all the fun. They got to run and get dirty and play without a shirt on. Boys played lots of sports and could be anything they wanted to be. Although my parents allowed, even encouraged, me to play sports and to be anything I wanted to be, society wasn't quite so open minded.

Nonetheless, I found a wonderful friend who became my husband who helped me go to medical school. Cultural norms foiled again! And we started a family and I found out that being a woman wasn't so bad. In fact, being a mother and taking part in life's greatest miracle, giving birth, was fabulous. And finally, I didn't want to be a boy anymore.

In fact, as I look back on my life, I find that some of the portraits that are painted most vividly on my memory are things surrounding my being a woman. And I suspect that most of my life experience has been influenced by my gender.

Being pregnant while I was in medical school didn't lend itself to a lot of time for introspection. But even in the hectic days of school I found myself pausing to wonder at the awesome process occurring inside my body. There was a new life growing there. And after my first child was born I would occasionally stop and look at this delightful child and be awestruck by the thought that my husband and I had created this life: it had grown inside me. This awe comes wafting back every time I am present at a delivery or wield the ultrasound wand allowing a mother to see the first outlines of the new life she is carrying. And I realize how especially lucky I am that I can relate to my patient in a way that less than half of the physicians can because I too have puffed up in pride and pleasure at the wonder of life in my womb. I cannot imagine that every physician who chooses to make maternity care a part of his or her practice does not have a bit of ongoing awe. But I am sorry for my male colleagues who can only look on because they can never have really been there!

Being a woman, and in this case a daughter, is part of another canvas as well. My mother died of lung cancer some years ago. Although being by her side as she lived her final days was painful, there was also a sharing, a deepening of our friendship that occurred. And her peace and grace in those last days showed me that with assistance of family, friends, and caring professionals, death can be embraced. It need not be ugly or terrifying. Over the years, this canvas, this collection of memories has helped me help many patients and their families through their own last days. Although this set of interactions is one that both men and women share, I am confident that the relationship between mother and daughter colors my recollections and my philosophies. Perhaps it has colored my own care patterns in the years that have followed.

*(continued)*

---

### Vignette (continued)

Now I have two daughters and the mother daughter relationship is being played out in the other direction. I delight that my daughters have grown up in a culture that allows girls to do virtually anything, when the glass ceilings and walls are coming down. I look forward to their progression through the many life stages that come to girls and women. And I relish the thought that there are many new experiences awaiting me as well, including grandparenting, weddings, and growing old and more dependent on those who currently depend on me.

I no longer wish I was a boy. I revel in the experiences that being a woman has brought me. Medicine is richer for having the perspective of both genders blended in the care and the caring and the curing.

*Nancy Dickey*

---

cal graduates in 1997 in the United States are (Pasko and Seidman 1999): internal medicine 23.1%, general/family practice 9.5%, pediatrics 9.1%, psychiatry 6.6%, anesthesiology 5.6%, general surgery 4.7%, obstetrics and gynecology 4.1%, pathology 3.3%. One study suggested that international medical graduates occupied the lowest prestige positions, male U.S. graduates the highest, and female U.S. graduates mid-level positions (Goldblatt & Goldblatt 1976). With a higher percentage of women among international medical graduates, their choices influence the statistics on women physicians.

---

*Women physicians average about a 50-hour workweek.*

---

## PRODUCTIVITY

Women physicians average more than a 40-hour workweek; in fact, it is more like a 50-hour workweek (Table 13-2). Women physicians worked about 89% as many hours per week as men physicians, and one less week per year. Thus, in the average year, women physicians averaged 2,435 hours, 87% of men physicians' 2,786 hours. Much of the difference in total hours can be attributed to more women practicing part-time. In one study (Hojat et al 1990), 17% of the women physicians, but only 3% of the men, worked part-time. The women physicians who worked full-time averaged 55 hours a week compared to men's 60 hours a week, whereas women and men working part-time averaged 33 and 34 hours (Hojat et al 1990). Women and men physician's work hours have become more similar over the years (Table 13-3).

Women work fewer hours at least partially because of children. Both men and women with young children work fewer hours (Lee and Mroz 1991), although the effect for women is typically greater than for men.

TABLE 13-2.
HOURS WORKED AND INCOME OF WOMEN AND MEN PHYSICIANS

|  | Women Physicians (WPHS, 1993) | Women Physicians (AMA, 1997) | Men Physicians (AMA, 1997) |
|---|---|---|---|
| Clinical hours worked per week | 36.8 | 48.0 | 54.2 |
| Nonclinical hours worked per week | 10.5 | 4.6 | 4.7 |
| Total professional hours worked per week | 47.3 | 52.6 | 58.9 |
| Total visits per week |  | 94.8 | 113.6 |
| Weeks worked per year |  | 46.3 | 47.3 |
| Mean annual income | $109,000 | $120,000 | $175,000 |

Source: Adapted from Frank et al 1997; Gonzalez ML, AMA data at http://www.ama-assn .org/advocacy/healthpolicy/x-ama/gender.htm

TABLE 13-3.
WOMEN PHYSICIAN'S WORK HOURS (PER WEEK) AS A PERCENTAGE OF
MEN PHYSICIAN'S WORK HOURS

| Study Author | Year | Percentage |
|---|---|---|
| Dykman and Stalnaker | 1953 | 71 |
| Heins et al | 1976 | 88 |
| Bobula | 1978 | 84 |
| Mattera | 1978 | 92 |
| Mitchell | 1978–79* | 98 |
| Silberger et al | 1986* | 91 |
| Gonzalez | 1997 | 89 |

These studies are not directly comparable and provide only a general overview of productivity.
*Physicians working less than 20 hours per week are excluded.

*American workers are working longer and harder than 20 years ago.*
*In surveys by the Families and Work Institute, a nonprofit research*
*group in New York, hours worked at all jobs for all employees*
*averaged 46 per week in 1998, up from 44 in the 1977 survey.*
*(Himmelberg M. Workers wonder: what became of the 8-hour day?*
Philadelphia Inquirer, *October 22, 1998, C1,C8.)*

Hours of work also differ by family income. According to Lee and Mroz (1991), physicians worked fewer hours when they had higher family incomes. Women physicians were more likely to have high family incomes (because they are more likely to have high-earning spouses, such as physicians, and more likely to have working spouses), and were more likely to reduce work hours. However, women were more likely to reduce their hours more in relationship to the same nonpractice income. Higher family income may be associated with physician husbands, particularly surgeons, whose long work hours may mean the woman physician spouse works more hours at home.

---

*Parenthood increased the productivity of employees, according to Carol Kleiman (Parenthood increases productivity, those who should know say.* Philadelphia Inquirer, *June 5, 2000, D4). The information was gleaned from a 1999 national survey of employed parents by the Lutheran Brotherhood, a nonprofit financial services organization based in Minneapolis.*

---

## INCOME

Women physicians earn a good income, averaging about $120,000 (Table 13-2). This is 69% of what men physicians make, which is about $175,000. These ratios are similar to what women make compared to men in the United States. Per hour, women physicians make about $49. This is 78% of what men physicians make, which is about $63. Some of the yearly income difference is based on the numbers of hours worked per week. Based on total visits per year, women physicians make 84% of what men do—$27.33 per visit compared to men's $32.57 per visit. Although this may seem unfair, much or most of the difference can be accounted for by different specialty choices as well as other factors:

- Specialty—women are much less likely to be in surgical specialties, which average much higher incomes, and more likely to be in primary care, which averages lower incomes. Men are almost four times as likely to be surgeons than women are. In addition, women are more likely to spend more time in primary care even when only a portion of what they do is primary care (Gonzalez). Overall, women physicians spend an average of 41% of their time, and men physicians 30% of their time, in primary care activities (Gonzalez).

- Employment status—self-employed physicians usually earn more [median income $200,000 compared to $140,000 (Gonzalez)]. Note that this difference between self-employed and employed physicians is about the same difference as that in the income between women and men physicians. In 1997, about 39% of women physicians and about 60% of men physicians were self-employed (Table 13-4).

- Patient payment status—women physicians have a higher percentage of earnings from managed care (49% compared to 43%) (Gonzalez). Managed care tends to pay less than traditional insurance. Women physicians

---

*Women physicians make less money than men physicians mostly because of specialty choices, practice type, and hours of work.*

---

were also more likely to have a higher percent of patients covered by Medicaid (about 17% compared to about 11%) (Gonzalez), which is traditionally low-paying. Women physicians have a higher percent of patients from low-income families (31% compared to 21%) and are more likely to practice in underserved locations (30% compared to 18%) (Hojat et al 1990).

- Age—as women are entering medicine in increasing numbers, their average age is lower than men physicians. However, peak earning occurs at about age 36 to 45. In 1997, 46% of women physicians were between 36 and 45, as were 33% of men physicians (Gonzalez). Thus, currently, age as a factor in earnings would suggest higher pay for women physicians.

The bottom line is that the differences in income may be totally accounted for by these types of factors. Baker (1996) looked at young physicians (<45 years of age, 2 to 9 years in practice) and found no difference in hourly income when accounting for specialty (13 fields of practice), practice setting (10 settings), medical education [type of medical school (public or private, U.S. or foreign), ranking of the school, graduate degrees acquired other than an M.D., and the taking of a leave of absence during medical school], experience (total years of practice experience and years in current main practice), personal characteristics (age, race or ethnic group, marital status, and parenthood status), AMA membership, specialty-board status (although the same percentage of men and women are board certified), characteristics of the community (number of concurrent practices), and experience with malpractice claims. In fact, his model suggested women in general or family practice may actually earn slightly more than men.

---

*Differences between the earnings of men and women should be expected because women have less experience in their work than men, women choose to major in areas that pay less, and women choose careers that enable them to combine work and family. (Furchtgott-Roth D, Stolba C. American women aren't really so cheap.* Wall Street Journal, *November 20, 1998 pg A-24.)*

---

## OTHER PRACTICE CHARACTERISTICS

- Women physicians are less likely to belong to the American Medical Association: 27% of young women belong, compared to 39% of young men (Baker 1996).
- Women physicians have about the same rate of board certification (Baker 1996).

- Women physicians are less likely to be sued than men physicians (Baker 1996; Mitka 1991; Sloan et al 1989). In a survey of young physicians, 15% of women and 22% of men physicians have been sued (Baker 1996). Part of this is because women physicians are less likely to be surgeons and perform fewer procedures (Chambers and Campbell 1996; Ellsbury et al 1987; Ogle et al 1986).

## Career Satisfaction

In some ways, what's there not to love about being a physician? Physicians have jobs that can be intellectually stimulating, can improve the world, may be flexible, and may generate considerable income, generously expressed gratitude from patients, and high societal esteem. However, each of these positive aspects has a negative counterpart: medical practice may be tedious and repetitive, some patients maintain unhealthy behaviors no matter how frequently and sincerely we try to help them change, the threat of malpractice suits constantly looms, physician autonomy and incomes have been restricted by HMOs, and patients may make unreasonable demands at unreasonable hours.

Given all these competing variables, how satisfied are women physicians with their careers? The answer, happily, is very satisfied: 84% of women physicians say they are usually, almost always, or always satisfied with their careers (Frank et al 1999). However, 31% would maybe, probably, or definitely not choose to be a physician again and 38% would maybe, probably, or definitely prefer to change their specialty (Frank et al 1999). Women physicians have similar satisfaction to men physicians (Bates et al 1998; Haas et al 1998; Hojat et al 1990), specifically for overall practice, income, leisure time, autonomy in decision making, relationships with patients, and relationships with peers (Bates et al 1998). Men physicians are more worried about interactions with hospital administrators, the potential oversupply of physicians, and medical malpractice litigation than women physicians, who are more worried about having time for family (Hojat et al 1990).

Let's examine in more detail the WPHS findings on women physician's satisfaction with practice. Who was most satisfied? WPHS showed that, unsurprisingly, women physicians who had more work control, less work stress, a comfortable amount of work, four to six on call nights per month, less severe harassment histories, older age, and better mental health also reported higher levels of career satisfaction. Work control and career satisfaction were especially strongly associated: those who believed they were always or almost always in control of their work life were 11 times more likely to be satisfied with their careers than were those who perceived little control. Similar characteristics were associated with a desire to again become a physician if reliving one's life, and with satisfaction with specialty. Especially high satisfaction with one's specialty was reported by dermatologists, surgeons, ophthalmologists, psychiatrists, and anesthesiologists; general practitioners and general internists were particularly interested in specialty change. Figure 13-1 shows the relationships among the three outcome measures (satisfaction with career, desire to become

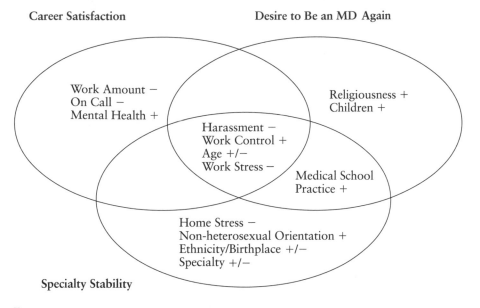

Career Satisfaction     Desire to Be an MD Again

Work Amount −
On Call −
Mental Health +

Religiousness +
Children +

Harassment −
Work Control +
Age +/−
Work Stress −

Medical School
Practice +

Home Stress −
Non-heterosexual Orientation +
Ethnicity/Birthplace +/−
Specialty +/−

**Specialty Stability**

FIGURE 13-1.
Overlapping variables in WPHS that predict career satisfaction, desire to again become a physician, and interest in changing one's specialty. The symbol (1) indicates that the variable has a positive relationship with the career satisfaction outcome with which it is associated; (2) indicates that the variable has a negative relationship with the outcome; and (1/2) indicates that it has positive relationships with some and negative relationships with others of the outcomes with which it is associated. Reprinted with permission from Arch Intern Med 1999, 159, 1417-26. © American Medical Association.

a physician again, and satisfaction with specialty choice) and the core variables: age, work control, work stress, and history of gender-based harassment.

Let's examine some of these variables in more detail, beginning with personal characteristics. For example, why would older physicians have greater career satisfaction? This may reflect generational differences in attitudes, expectations, and experiences; having attained a more senior, more satisfying job; a dimmed recall of training's rigors; or "pioneer pride." Or perhaps they no longer have children at home, which makes their lives seem more controllable and their careers more satisfying. The lesser likelihood of younger physicians wanting to change specialty may be attributable to the greater opportunities now available for women in historically male-dominated specialties from which prior women graduates may have been excluded.

What about the effect of children? Most literature on women physicians and children has focused on negative outcomes of multiple roles, such as role conflict and strain, but WPHS found that physicians with children were more interested in again becoming a physician, suggesting that having children may

TABLE 13-4.
TYPE OF PRIMARY PROFESSIONAL ACTIVITY OF WOMEN AND MEN
PHYSICIANS

|  | Women Physicians (%) (AMA, 1997) | Men Physicians (%) (AMA, 1997) |
| --- | --- | --- |
| Office-based practice | 54.9 | 63.2 |
| Hospital-based practice (full-time staff) | 13.5 | 11.3 |
| Resident/fellow | 14.2 | 8.9 |
| Administration | 1.1 | 1.3 |
| Medical teaching | 1.1 | 1.0 |
| Medical research | 1.3 | 1.7 |
| Other | 0.5 | 0.4 |
| Inactive | 6.0 | 6.7 |

Adapted from Pasko and Seidman 1999 with permission.

bring both personal and professional benefits, and some other studies have found this as well. This issue is discussed in more detail in Chapter 6.

Several professional factors were also found in WPHS to be associated with career satisfaction. Dermatologists, anesthesiologists, and psychiatrists may be more content due to work control factors such as fewer on-call demands and greater control of work hours. Surgeons may have especially strong "pioneer pride," or be more satisfied with higher income or particularly high control in their daily professional interactions. The higher dissatisfaction seen in general internists and radiologists is an especially important and potentially remediable target for intervention and further investigation. Radiologists' dissatisfaction seems especially remediable; they earned considerably more than did other women physicians but were also more likely to feel they worked too many hours. It can be very seductive to work too many hours, especially when one is very well paid for one's time.

In WPHS and in other studies, the strongest professional predictors of career satisfaction were control of work environment and work stress. Highly stressed individuals who feel they lack control may be at risk to leave the profession, change specialty, or be unhappily employed.

Practice site also was an important predictor of physician satisfaction in the WPHS (Table 13-4). Physicians practicing in medical schools were twice as likely as some other physicians to desire to become a doctor again and to be comfortable in their specialty, suggesting benefits from collegial and intellectually stimulating environments. Alternatively, it may suggest that doctors with especially firm convictions about their specialties and about medicine migrate toward academia. This has implications for medical students making decisions about specialty choices, as women physicians with whom they are in contact may be more satisfied than those in nonacademic practices.

Finally, WPHS also showed that having a history of gender-based or sexual harassment had serious negative effects on career satisfaction; this is discussed in Chapter 7.

What about comparisons with career satisfaction in other professionals? The two studies that shed light on this suggest that physicians may be more satisfied than nurses with income and professional interactions (Stamps et al 1978), and a comparable study of lawyers (Smith 1984) produced high percentages who seriously considered leaving the profession (27%).

Overall, women physicians are satisfied with their practices.

## ACKNOWLEDGMENTS

Julia E. McMurray, M.D., Mark Linzer, M.D., and Lisa Elon, M.P.H. participated in the data analysis of women physicians' career satisfaction, and contributed valuable insights into data interpretation.

## CHAPTER 14

# WOMEN PHYSICIANS AS HEALERS

MARJORIE A. BOWMAN AND ERICA FRANK

Women and men are different. Sociologic literature provides much evidence of difference. Women think differently (Belenky et al 1986; Gilligan 1982), have different bodies, conduct their lives differently, and have fewer leadership roles in organizations. Differences between individual men and women may vary, but the groups as a whole show some characteristic differences.

Simplistically, women physicians are women, and from this perspective may differ from men in their roles and actions in the health care system as healers or patients. Early sex-role orientations are highly reinforced (Weisman and Teitelbaum 1985; Williams and Best 1982), and resistant to change (Weisman and Teitelbaum 1985). Presuming that this means women physicians have more feminine characteristics than men physicians, how does being a woman influence how an individual practices medicine? Much of this book addressed systematic differences between groups of men and women physicians. Many believe that women bring humanism and caring to the profession of medicine. At least one author (Restak 1986) has gone so far as to declare, "We need more cheap, docile women doctors." What is the end result of the differences between men and women physicians? Is medical care cheaper? More humane? Are women physicians better healers than men physicians? This chapter brings together a variety of literature to provide some insight on women physicians as healers and patients.

# SEX-RELATED DIFFERENCES IN ACHIEVEMENT

Women physicians are less successful than men physicians by classical (male) definitions: they earn less money per hour, see fewer patients, have less academic success, and have less position power (i.e., leadership positions in organizations). In thinking about why this might be, there are five major theories: lower ability, less achievement motivation, lower confidence, personality differences, and discrimination.

## Ability

Physicians are a highly selected group. They are from the select group that goes to college, and then from the group selected from high college achievers that go to medical school.

There are those who think that men and women in the general population have differences in ability, such as with verbal or quantitative ability. However, the difference is about 1% of the variance for verbal and 4% for quantitative ability (Jacklin 1981). A genetic hypothesis has not been confirmed for differences in quantitative ability through direct tests, possibly because of differential feedback given to girls and boys throughout school (Jacklin 1981).

However, the literature on sex-related differences in ability is fraught with methodological problems. Jacklin (1981) identified several major ones, including problems with definition of "difference," confusion about statistically significant versus sufficient size effect, bias toward publishing studies showing differences, lack of control for differences in self-report by men and women (with men more defensive in self-reporting and less likely to disclose personal feelings), problems of within-sex versus between sex differences, nongeneralizable samples, and the large number of variables potentially confounded with sex. She notes that the better the sex-related research, the less sex has been found to account for variance in characteristics or behaviors. We believe her conclusions could be applied to inherent sex-related differences between men and women physicians today. In fact, similar types of problems are found in much research.

Even if a 10% difference were found, it would mean that 90% is the same. This means more within-group variability than between-group variability. Women and men have similar, though slightly different, scores on national tests, as outlined in Chapter 12.

## Achievement Motivation

Men are believed to be more likely to attribute outcome to their ability and consider their ability higher regardless of success or failure; women are believed to be more likely to attribute outcome to luck (Frieze et al 1982). Although metaanalysis of multiple studies confirmed these gender links (Frieze et al 1982), the differences were small and the authors noted that some studies were contradictory. In one study not included in the metaanalysis, men attending local fairs were more likely to choose games requiring skill and to persist longer, whereas women chose games involving luck (Deaux et al 1975), perhaps because of men's greater confidence in their own abilities. In another study (Feather 1969), which looked at expectations, unexpected success was more attributed to luck and associated with greater satisfaction for both genders. However, the female subjects were lower in confidence and higher in perceived inadequacy than male subjects and were more likely to attribute success or failure to luck.

Another way to consider confidence and achievement motivation is to determine how men and women view other men's and women's abilities, called attribution studies. Men are expected to be more successful (Feldman-Summers and Kiesler 1974), and undergraduate subjects rated successful female physicians as more motivated than successful male physicians (Feldman-Summers and Kiesler 1974). Male and female mental health therapists held similar concepts for healthy adults and healthy men but had a different concept for healthy adults and healthy women (Broverman et al 1970). When subjects were asked to rate the performance of males and females on male- or female-related tasks, subjects believed the males to be more skillful in either male- or female-related tasks, and the performance of the males to be more related to skill overall on the male task (Deaux and Emswiller 1974). In considering a male or female failing an exam for three sex-linked occupations (medicine, teaching, and nursing), female subjects downgraded successful females in relationship to unsuccessful females but upgraded successful males in relationship to unsuccessful males regardless of the three occupations (Feather and Simon 1975). Overall, successful males or successful females were rated higher than either the unsuccessful males or unsuccessful females and males were given more credit for success and females more blame for failure. Thus, attribution studies suggest that females should desire less success, as they will be blamed more for failure and receive less recognition for success.

## Confidence

Women are generally less confident in achievement settings, but this is probably dependent on the actual situation (Lenney 1977). Women are more likely to be confident with "feminine" tasks than with "masculine" tasks, even when the sex definitions have been manipulated (Lenney 1977). Women are more likely to have more confidence when given clear feedback (Lenney 1977). Lower confidence translates into choosing less demanding tasks, giving up more easily in the setting of failure (Lenney 1977), and having lower chances of success (Feather 1969).

Lower self-confidence is at least partially socially determined. Women are less confident in a social environment but not when they work alone or do not expect their performance to be compared to that of others (Lenney 1977). Hoffman (1972) agrees with this and argues that socialization encourages affiliation (i.e., development of social relationships) in young girls, and, if achievement threatens affiliation, girls will sacrifice performance or experience anxiety. In other words, relationships are more important than achievement for women, leading to less self-confidence and less achievement motivation.

Women professional students also see themselves as more feminine than the ideal practitioner in their field (Coplin and Williams 1978; Davis et al 1984; Giles and Williams 1979), speculatively leading to more anxiety about role performance.

## The Evidence in Medicine

The profession of medicine would appear to be a sex-linked area ("male") with high social interaction and unclear feedback on performance. Thus, the cited literature suggests that women physicians would (1) be lower in confidence, (2) be less willing to choose high-demand situations or those tasks considered "masculine," and (3) face more anxiety over their performance. At least partially as a result of these characteristics, they would be less successful.

In fact, the evidence in medicine, though limited in quantity and quality, suggests these hypotheses to be true. For example, women with mediocre performance in college are less like to apply and, ultimately, get into medical school than men with similarly mediocre performances (Fiorentine 1987). Noncognitive variables are more predictive of women's performance in medical school, whereas cognitive variables are more predictive for men (Willoughby et al 1979). Women are still less likely to choose traditional male specialties or male tasks and perform fewer procedures in practice (Bensing et al 1993; Ellsbury et al 1987; Ogle et al 1986). They feel less prepared for practice, particularly in surgical areas (Ellsbury et al 1987) and less confident in their diagnoses (Bensing et al 1993). There is no literature on specific attributions for success of women physicians. On the other hand, at least one study suggests that the level of confidence of women physicians may improve from the time of entry to medical school to a follow-up 8 to 10 years later (Cartwright 1972). And, as seen already, women are less successful in medicine by traditional measurements.

## Personality Differences

The major method of considering differences between men and women is sex-role typing. The Bem Sex-Role Inventory is a widely known instrument assessing traits frequently attributed to each sex. Masculine traits are described by such adjectives as aggressive, assertive, ambitious, competitive, and dominant. Adjectives for female traits include compassionate, understanding, sensitive to the needs of others, and yielding. It is often said that the same characteristic seen as positive for men are viewed as negative for women—assertiveness in men is good and in women it is bad. This has been borne out in the literature; for example, in one study (Butler and Geis 1990), female leaders who offered the same suggestions and arguments as male leaders were more negatively rated by the group (of men and women).

## Vignette

As AMA staff, I have observed certain "truths" about women physicians over the years. They always excel but rarely talk about it. What they accomplish in any given hour, day, or year is truly amazing. Yet, like many women, they are often reticent about valuing and selling those strengths and accomplishments. Another observation: Having extended many invitations to women physicians to serve on committees, present at meetings, or testify at hearings, I am usually met with these immediate responses: "How much time will it take?" and "I'm really not an expert." These are seldom issues for their male counterparts. It's a curious thing.

*Phyllis Kopriva*

In general women score higher on feminine characteristics and men on masculine characteristics, with a third category being androgynous (high on both masculine and feminine behaviors), and a fourth being undifferentiated (low on both masculine and feminine behaviors) (Hoffman and Fidell 1979). Other terms are used to describe the differences: independent/instrumental/scientific/reserved/technical versus affiliative/expressive/interpersonal/helping oriented/humane. These sex stereotypes had changed very little in the United States in the 16 years prior to 1980 (Williams and Best 1982). The masculine profile tends to be valued more in our society (Broverman et al 1972), probably because of higher levels of activity and strength in the definition (Best et al 1980). Women do not see themselves as less "good" (Williams and Best 1982), just less "strong" and "active" (Best et al 1980).

It could be theorized that androgyny would be the best sex-role type for physicians, because physicians are expected to be independent and assertive yet responsive to the needs of others (Shapiro et al 1983); i.e., a physician should combine the good aspects of both sexual stereotypes. The ideal physician is considered more androgynous than the ideal lawyer (compare Giles and Williams 1979 and Coplin and Williams 1978). Medical students conceive of their ideal physician as androgynous (Giles and Williams 1979); very similar findings held true for physician assistant students as well (Davis et al 1984). Also, both male and female androgynous individuals, followed by masculine individuals, have more self-esteem and less neuroticism than feminine or undifferentiated individuals (Hoffman and Fidell 1979), another potential advantage of androgyny for physicians. Individuals tend to describe the ideal sex-role traits as at the androgynous level (Williams and Best 1982), and those who are androgynous are more flexible behaviorly, which would appear to have advantages for mental health. Consistent with this, Clark and Zeldow (1988) found that higher masculinity was associated with less depression for male medical students, and women who were more aggressive, worldly, or not easily hurt had less depression. These differences in self-esteem and implied advantages for androgyny, however, do not clearly translate into differences in the health of the different sex-role types (Hoffman and Fidell 1979).

There is little information available in the literature on sex-role types of physicians. Williams and Best (1982) found women medical students to rate themselves as about the same in femininity as typical female college students but more feminine than the ideal physician (Giles and Williams 1979). The ideal physician was considered to be androgynous. Because female medical students rated themselves as further from the ideal, i.e., more feminine (Giles and Williams 1979), the female students could have more anxiety over their performance. Similarly, female physician-assistant students (Davis et al 1984) and law students (Coplin and Williams 1978) rated themselves as more feminine than the ideal person in their profession. Shapiro et al (1983) found that female patients considered female physicians to be more androgynous, less masculine, and more feminine than male physicians. There were no significant differences in the rating of the male and female physicians by male patients. Male medical students and male physicians saw female physicians as much more feminine and male physicians as much more masculine. Female medical students saw female physicians as more androgynous. Overall, women physicians were seen more as androgynous by patients and men physicians as undifferentiated. The authors conclude that male and female physicians are considered different from each other, but that the extent and type of differences are variable, depending on who rated them.

Several studies, which have discussed various aspects of the personalities of men and women physicians using techniques other than traditional sex-role measures, in general confirm the sex-role typing of women physicians as possessing more feminine traits than men physicians. Several have found that women students are more attuned to patient relationships. For example, Cartwright (1972) found first-year women students had more sensitivity to relationships and more general acceptance of feelings than men students. Bergquist et al (1985) found women medical students placed more value on patient contact. Women medical student applicants (Roessler et al 1975) scored higher on nurturing, change, impulsivity, understanding, and harm avoidance, and lower on dominance, exhibition, and order scales. The accepted and rejected women medical students were not different. In a longitudinal survey, Leserman (1981) found new women students placed more value on psychosocial factors in health care. In an interesting twist on this question, Gross and Crovitz (1975) asked medical students to rate women medical students versus other women on different categories; the women medical students were rated to be as nurturing as women but more aggressive, exacting, enduring, achievement oriented, intellectual, and dominant than women in the general population.

With the Myers-Briggs Scale, Rezler and Buckley (1977) found that women medical students in general were guided more than other women health care professional students by thinking than by feelings in their approach to work and other people. Unfortunately, the authors did not have comparison male students. Within each group, there were marked differences among the students. In

contrast, Maheux et al (1988) reported the professional and sociopolitical attitudes of 343 female and 380 male medical students from a northwestern state
in 1979 to be similar, with increasing similarity at more advanced levels of
training.

Crowson et al (1986) considered health locus of control of 21 men and 13
women internal medicine residents. This is a measure of the extent to which
the individual perceives control of the results of his/her own behavior; for example, external locus of control suggests that luck explains what happens to
an individual, whereas internal locus of control suggests that the person is responsible for his/her behavior. Crowson et al (1986) found the women had a
greater external locus of control ($p < .001$); however, Frey et al (1981) had
found no difference in a similar study of family practice first-year residents.
There have been no larger studies comparing locus of control or elucidating
the full implications of locus of control for physicians.

Lorber (1984) found that men and women physicians similarly described
the patients they liked best and least. Of the women and men physicians she
interviewed, only one woman physician believed that women handled patients
differently. However, when asked about their accomplishments in medicine,
the women were more likely to discuss the personal or caring aspect, and men
their therapeutic skills, consistent with typical sex-role typing. Women also
value the psychosocial aspects of care higher than men (Hojat et al 1995).
Women physicians may relate better to dying patients, finding it easier to discuss death and console families (Dickinson and Pearson 1979).

## The Evidence: Differences in Practice

There are some differences in practice styles between women and men
physicians. In particular, women physicians see more women patients,
do more prevention, and spend more time with each patient, although
the gender differences are small. Quality of care appears to be similar,
and women and men physicians treat comparable patients similarly but
have different types of patients (women physicians have more female and
young patients). Women patients disclose more to women physicians,
particularly for mental health, personal, or sexually related concerns.
Women physicians are sued less frequently.

### More Women Patients

First and foremost, a fact on which all authors agree, women physicians see
more women patients (see Chapter 7) (Bensing et al 1993; Britt et al 1996;
Hartzema and Christensen 1983). Not only do female physicians see more
women, they are more likely to see women specifically for genitourinary types

of problems, and provide more endocrine care (Bensing et al 1993, Britt et al 1996).

### More Prevention Services

Female physicians value prevention and nutrition more than male physicians (Hojat et al 1995; Lurie et al 1997; Maheux et al 1990). Physicians report more comfort with same-sex sexual histories and examinations (Lurie et al 1998). The following studies have also found that women physicians offer and complete more prevention services with their patients, including counseling:

- Franks and Clancy (1993), based on National Ambulatory Medical Care Survey (NAMCS) data, difference found in Pap smears and mammograms but not blood pressure checks
- Ewing et al (1999), self-reported data from a survey of 3,881 primary care clinicians
- Levy et al (1992), patients over age 50, chart audit
- Frank and Harvey (1996), self-reported data
- Kreuter et al (1995)
- Lurie et al (1993), from insurance claims for Pap smears and mammography
- Majeroni et al (1993), chart review
- Hall et al (1990), chart audit
- Seto et al (1996), hormone replacement therapy

None of these studies accounted fully for differences in types of patients. Nor does the sex of the physician account for most of the inadequate compliance with national prevention guidelines.

In 1977, the National Ambulatory Medical Care Survey (NAMCS 80-1710) compared selected diagnostic services ordered or provided with the sex of the physicians. "The only statistically significant result showed that female physicians were more likely to check blood pressure during visits for symptoms referring to the genitourinary system than were men." Women physicians did more blood pressure checks and Pap tests, probably reflective of different patient populations. Proportionately more new patients were seen by the women, but men physicians saw more patients on referral than women. When asked to judge the seriousness of the patient's condition, men physicians believed their patients to be more seriously ill.

In the 1980c–81c NAMCS survey (NAMCS 84-1737), female obstetrician-gynecologists were more likely than their male counterparts to have new patients and to use Pap tests, laboratory tests, blood pressure checks, and diet counseling during visits. The female general and family practitioners ordered more Pap tests and clinical laboratory tests and provided more medical counseling (NAMCS 1980a–81a, 83-1734). Female pediatricians used general history and/or examination more frequently and had a higher proportion of visits that included blood pressure checks, diet counseling, and family or social counseling (84-1737). Some of the differences could be attributed to differences in patient populations, with women physicians having more new patients, women, and younger patients.

## More Time with Patients
Women physicians spend more time with their patients. The 1977 NAMCS survey (NAMCS 80-1710) reported that "the mean duration of all visits to women specialists was 17.8 minutes, compared with 15.3 to male specialists, which was chiefly due to the average time used by general and family practitioners (17.6 minutes for females in this specialty, compared to 12.7 minutes for males in the practice)." Similarly, longer duration visits were found in NAMCS for general and family practitioners (NAMCS 83-1734), pediatricians (NAMCS 1980b–81b, 84-1736) and ob/gyns (NAMCS 84-1737). Part or all of these differences could results from increased preventive and counseling services. Roter et al (1991) reported that female primary care physicians averaged 22.9 minutes per encounter compared to male physicians' 20.3 minutes; both the patients and physicians talked more in the female physician encounters. Similar time differences were found for Dutch general practitioners (Bensing et al 1993) and pediatricians (Bernzweig et al 1997).

## Skill
There are few data on the skill of female physicians. One study by Schueneman et al (1985) found that women surgery residents (13 women representing 10% of the total in the study) were academically more qualified than the men and did better on a visual perception task, but scored less well on a perceptual task involving both motor analysis and visual analysis in psychometric testing (which relates to operative skill) and were rated less well by their surgical superiors. The authors attributed this lower rating to potentially greater cautiousness in avoiding errors and also noted that supervisors rate females less well in the area of confidence and task organization. The authors also quote another study (McGee 1979) that found men to be more spatially and motor proficient than women, although the author does not specify the amount of difference between the sexes. Although this is a small number of women from which to generalize and there was very little difference between the men and women, this could suggest a complex mixture of effects creating a lack of confidence in surgical skills, including greater cautiousness on the part of women in performing motor skills, and contributing to less confidence in the training setting reinforced by generally male superiors.

## More Disclosure/Psychosocial Care
Patients may be more likely to disclose mental illness symptoms or personal concerns to same-sex physicians (Young 1979). In reviewing the literature on disclosure of symptoms to physicians, Young (1979) noted that there was inconsistency in results but believed that the major reason for this was the studies had not taken into account what type of symptoms were to be disclosed. When the type of symptoms was determined, as in Young's study, greater disclosure to same-sex physician became more apparent. An alternative explana-

tion for inconsistency in this literature is the year the study was done and the experience rate of patients with male and female physicians. As fewer patients in earlier studies would have had the opportunity to see women physicians, their reaction may have been less positive (Engleman 1974). The concept of greater disclosure to same-sex physicians is reinforced by studies that have found that people will divulge more feelings to same-sex individuals in situations other than doctor-patient relationships (Highlen and Gillis 1978). In a study of Dutch general practitioners, both male and female patients were more likely to see female physicians for "social" problems (Bensing et al 1993); similarly, female Australian general practitioners were more likely to see patients for psychosocial problems (Britt et al 1996). Women physicians value interpersonal skills, psychological and social factors in health, and ethical issues more highly than men physicians (Hojat et al 1995). When a patient simulated minor depression, women physicians were far more likely to recommend counseling, and both men and women physicians recommended counseling more often when the patient was a woman rather than a man (Badger et al 1999). The men physicians were also more likely to recommend antidepressants to the women portraying minor depression than to the men, whereas women physicians prescribed at similar rates for men and women.

In another study (Riessman 1979), women were more likely to disclose to male interviewers presumed to be lower status, and men to those of higher status. Similarly, Levinson et al (1984) found that men more strongly desired men physicians than women wanted women physicians, though both tended to want same-sex physicians, and that emotional problems or medical problems that required greater physical intimacy (complete physical exam, gynecologic or prostate problem) also produced higher desires for same-sex physicians.

For genetic counseling, a female provider (not specifically physician) was better for female patients. When there was a female provider, there were more in-depth discussion and clearer explanations, and female patients were more likely to disclose concerns, although the counseling sessions were similar in length (Zare et al 1984).

In a survey study of women physicians, Dickinson and Pearson (1979) found that women physicians tended to relate better to dying patients and their families and to become more depressed when a patient died.

## More Partnership Building

Women physicians spent more time talking with patients, providing more information and building partnerships. The patients asked more questions, and there was more positive talk between women physicians and their patients in a study that rated actual doctor-patient communication (Roter et al 1991). Hall et al (1994) confirmed this in a study that found women physicians provided more emotional support, partnership building, and positive talk. A study of pediatricians (Bernzweig et al 1997) similarly found more communication with children. In another way to consider this, West (1993) found that men physicians were more likely to give explicit commands to their patients ("Just take one four times a day"), whereas women physicians were more likely to use less direct statements, which could be seen as proposals ("Let's talk about your pressure for a minute or two." "Well, let's make that our plan."). Probably as a result, women physicians achieved a higher rate of responses of adherence from the patients.

## Other

Other aspects of medical care or diagnoses have been considered. Female pediatricians in NAMCS (84-1737) prescribed drugs more frequently, although this had not been found to be true in the 1977 survey (NAMCS 80-1710) or for the ob-gyns (NAMCS 84-1737) or general and family practitioners (NAMCS 83-1734), or in the Dutch general practitioner study (Bensing et al 1993). Similarly, Hartzema and Christensen (1983) found physician sex did not explain differences in drug prescribing behavior when other factors were taken into account.

In the Dutch general practitioner study (Bensing et al 1993), female physicians ordered more laboratory tests (however, diagnosis was not taken into account, and it is not clear if this included Pap smears).

Another study compared medical workups by 10 male and 10 female physicians in a health maintenance organization for 142 male and 165 female patients with chief complaints of chest pain, headache, dizziness, fatigue, and back pain, and found no difference in the extent of the workup or the appropriateness of the workup based on the sex of the physician or patient (Greer et al 1986). The treatment of menorrhagia also does not vary with the sex of the physician (Coulter et al 1995).

Women ob/gyns were more likely to strongly believe that women should have the right to abortions and were more likely to believe that federal funds should pay for abortions (Weisman et al 1986). Women ob/gyns were also more likely to perform abortions but averaged fewer abortions per provider. Women ob/gyns were less likely to provide amniocentesis and artificial inseminations and some other infertility services (Weisman et al 1987). In a more recent study in Canada, Bouchard and Renaud (1997) found that women physicians were more liberal in their attitudes about providing access to amniocentesis and selective abortion and had a less directive relationship with their patients.

Women physicians are sued less frequently (Medica 1983; Mitka 1991; Sloan et al 1989), probably because they perform fewer procedures (Chambers and Campbell 1996; Ellsbury et al 1987; Ogle et al 1986) and possibly because of better doctor-patient relationships.

## SUMMARY

In general, men and women physicians perform similar medical workups for similar types of patients, whereas women physicians spend longer time with each patient, provide more preventive care, and have more women patients. Data suggest that there is greater disclosure in same-sex doctor-patient relationships, which should lead to better care, but that is unproven.

Same-sex dyads would be most likely to help when patients state a preference for the sex of their physician; when sexual, mental health, or personal symptoms are treated; or when significant doctor-patient negotiation is required. However, in individual circumstances, the potential improvement could easily be outbalanced by other important factors such as access, skill, or other personal and professional characteristics.

Women physicians are generally less confident, or perhaps, said a different way, feel less strong and active, or less motivated to achieve. There is little research to suggest the impact of this on quality of care. It could mean more attention is taken in thinking through patients' problems, which should improve outcome. Less risk taking lowers malpractice risk and decreases the risk to the patient, but could mean less gain for patients for whom the risk would have paid off. It may mean that the patient, in detecting the lower confidence, feels less secure, and thus is less readily cured through the placebo qualities of the doctor-patient relationship. It certainly means that women are less likely to strive for organizational and administrative leadership roles.

Many of the differences between men and women are socially reinforced. It would seem that social reinforcement of the differences between the sexes serves the functioning of society in some manner. Reinforcing differences between male and female physicians can also be positive, offering different opportunities for patients to maximize their own wishes in choice of physician.

On the whole, women and women physicians as compared to men and men physicians are (1) more oriented to relationships, with men more oriented to procedures; (2) more feminine or androgynous; (3) less confident in their abilities with equivalent training and intelligence; and (4) less motivated to achieve by traditional measures. Overall, women physicians are more different among themselves than between themselves and men physicians. Said another way, women physicians are similar to men physicians but retain many characteristics attributed to women in our society (Weisman and Teitelbaum 1985). Both men and women physicians represent subgroups of their sexes with some generalizable characteristics and much internal variability. Women offer much to medicine and may be the physicians of choice for many patients and situations.

## PREDICTIONS

What can be predicted? Women are an increasing percentage of physicians, and have increased their numbers in traditional male specialties. There are slight increases in leadership positions. We believe the differences cited above have persisted throughout our professional lives and are likely to continue. As Helen Fisher (2000) said (author of *The First Sex: The Natural Talents of Women and How They are Changing the World*), women are more interested in balancing work and family. Her prediction? "Physicians who use high-tech medicine will be men, whereas women will practice more hands-on medicine."

## CHAPTER 15

# CONCLUSIONS

MARJORIE A. BOWMAN

Women physicians are an increasing proportion of the profession. Attitudes are changing, and there is considerable improvement in the place and role of women in medicine. Women physicians are happy in their careers and lives and thus are successful on their own terms, although they do hold far fewer positions of power, make less money, and advance in academic careers more slowly than men—all traditional (male) indicators of success. Although women comprise close to half of medical students, it will be many years before the physician population is half women. The increasing numbers, however, should help junior women find role models and like-minded supporters with whom to share experiences and gain insight.

Has medicine become more humane because of the increasing percentage and numbers of women physicians? We would like to think so. In fact, as compared to the data available at the time of the first two editions of this book, it is increasingly obvious that women physicians do make a difference. Unmistakably, women patients often prefer women physicians. Women physicians practice exemplary personal health practices and encourage similarly high levels of prevention in their patients. Women patients with women physicians are more likely to discuss psychological or sexual issues. These attributes of women physicians are in and of themselves excellent. But, in addition, we believe that women physicians in leadership positions could bring a more participatory style of management and increasing attention to minority and poor patients, a theory that we would like to see tested by the advancement of women into the highest positions of leadership!

Women physicians also struggle. Juggling careers, families, and personal time is serious work and takes thoughtful, ongoing efforts and varying strategies over a lifetime. We are real people who must face career setbacks, mistakes, sickness, abuse/violence, family disappointments, divorce, and death. Physicians have great responsibility and confront many ethical, monetary, and major, frequently urgent, medical decisions. Our role in society remains generally exalted and highly paid. In general we handle these potentially conflicting challenges and rewards with aplomb, but there are many times we need the solace of friends, fellow physicians, families, and supportive persons of many varieties, including mental health professionals, and must call on every stress-management technique we can imagine.

We admit we need help. We hire help. We turn to each other. We love, we share, we give, we learn, and we help others. Ours is a caring profession for which we sacrifice much and from which we gain much. We are rightfully proud of our fellow women physicians and continue to be awed by all they do, and by how well they do it.

# REFERENCES

## CHAPTER 1

ABRAM RJ. Send us a lady physician: women doctors in America 1835–1920. W. W. Norton, New York, 1985.

AMA. Physician characteristics and distribution in the US. American Medical Education, Chicago, 1999.

BICKEL J, CROFT K, MARSHALL R. Women in U.S. academic medicine statistics 1998. Association of American Medical Colleges, Washington, DC, 1998.

BROWN CA. Women workers in the health service industry. Int J Health Serv 1975; 5(2):173–184.

BULLOUGH V, VOGHT M. Women, menstruation and nineteenth century medicine. Bull Hist Med 1973; 47:66–82.

FIDELL LA. Sex role stereotypes and the American physician. Psychol Wom Q 1980; 4(3):313–330.

HEINS M. Women physicians: they've come a long way, but what of the future? Radcliffe Q June 1979; 11–14.

MORANTZ-SANCHEZ RM. Sympathy and science: women physicians in American medicine. Oxford University Press, New York, 1985.

NADELSON C. The woman physician: past, present and future. In: Callan JP, ed. The physician—a professional under stress. Appleton-Century-Crofts, Norwalk, CT, 1983: 261–276.

SHYROCK RH. Medicine in America: historical essays. Johns Hopkins University Press, Baltimore, 1966: 184.

TURNER TB. Women in medicine—a historical perspective. J Am Med Wom Assoc 1981; 36(2)33–37.

WALSH MR. Doctors wanted: no women need apply. Yale University Press, New Haven and London, 1977.

# CHAPTER 2

BLACKWELL B. Prevention of impairment among residents in training. JAMA 1986; 255:1177–1178.

BROWN JB. Female family doctors: their work and well-being. Fam Med 1992; 24:591–595.

CAMPBELL MA. Why would a girl go into medicine? Feminist Press, New York, 1973.

CARTWRIGHT LIC. Role montage: life patterns of professional women. J Am Med Wom Assoc 1987; 42(5):142–148.

CHARLES SC, WARNECKE RB, WILBERT JR, LICHTENBERG R, DEJESUS C. Sued and non-sued physicians: satisfactions, dissatisfactions, and sources of stress. Psychomatics 1987; 28(9):462–466.

CHERNISS C. Professional burnout in human service organizations. Praeger, New York, 1980:41.

CHROUSOS GP, GOLD PW. The concepts of stress and stress system disorders: overview of physical and behavioral homeostasis. JAMA 1992; 267:1244–1252.

COBURN D, JOVAISAS AV. Perceived sources of stress among first year medical students. J Med Educ 1975; 50:589–595.

COECK C, LORENS PG, VANDEVIVERE J, MAHLER C. ACTH and cortisol levels during residency training. N Engl J Med 1991; 325:738.

COHEN F, KEMENY ME, KEARNEY KA, et al. Persistent stress as a predictor of genital herpes recurrence. Arch Intern Med 1999; 159:2430–2436.

COHEN M, WOODWARD CA, FERRIER BM. Factors influencing career development: do men and women differ? *J Am Med Wom Assoc* 1988; 43:142–154.

COLFORD JM, MCPHEE SJ. Ravelled sleeve of care. JAMA 1989; 261:889–893.

DAVIDSON K, JONAS BS, DIXON KE, MARKOVITZ JH. Do depression symptoms predict early hypertension incidence in young adults in the CARDIA study? Arch Intern Med 2000; 160:1495–1500.

FORD ES, AHLUWALIA IB, GALUSKA DA. Social relationships and cardiovascular disease risk factors: findings from the Third National Health and Nutrition Examination Survey. Prev Med 2000; 30:83–92.

FRIEDMAN RC, KORNFIELD DS, BIGGER TJ. Psychological problems associated with sleep deprivation in interns. J Med Educ 1973;48:436–441.

GLASER R, RABIN B, CHESNEY M, COHEN S, NATELSON B. Stress-induced immunomodulation: implications for infectious diseases? JAMA 1999; 281:2268–2270.

GOTTHEIL E, THORNTON CC, CONLY SS, CORNELISON FS JR. Stress, satisfaction, and performance: transition from university to medical college. J Med Educ 1969; 44:270–277.

GROSS EB. Gender differences in physician stress: why the discrepant findings? Women & Health 1997; 26(3):1–14.

HALERAN JF. Doctors don't have to burn out. Med Econ 1981; Oct 26:148–161.

JOHNSON JV, HALL EM. Job strain, workplace social support, and cardiovascular disease: a cross-sectional study of a random sample of the Swedish working population. Am J Public Health 1988; 78:1336–1342.

JOHNSON JV, HALL EM, FORD DE, et al. The psychosocial work environment of physicians. J Occup Environ Med 1995; 37:1151–1159.

KARASEK R, BAKER D, MARXER F, AHLBOM A, THEORELL T. Job decision latitude, job demands, and cardiovascular disease: a prospective study of Swedish men. Am J Public Health 1981; 71:694–705.

KELLNER R, WIGGING RG, PATHAK D. Hypochondrical fears and beliefs in medical and law students. Arch Gen Psychiatry 1986; 43(5):487–489.

KING M, STANLEY G, BURROWS G. Stress: theory and practice. Gram & Stratton, Orlando, FL 1987.

KRANTZ DS, SHEPS DS, CARNEY RM, NATELSON BH. Effects of mental stress in patients with coronary artery disease. JAMA 2000; 283:1800–1802.

LA ROSA JH. Women, work, and health: employment as a risk factor for coronary heart disease. Am J Obstet Gynecol 1988; 158:1597–1602.

LAMBERG L. "If I worked hard(er), I will be loved." Roots of physician stress explored. JAMA 1999; 282:13–14.

LURIE N, RANK B, PARENTI C, et al. How do house officers spend their nights? N Engl J Med 1989; 320:1673–1677.

McCALL TB. The Libby Zion case. N Engl J Med 1988;318:771–778.

McCUE JD. The effects of stress on physicians and their medical practice. N Engl J Med 1982; 306:458–476.

McKEGNEY CP. Medical education: a neglectful and abusive family system. Fam Med 1989; 21:452–457.

MURPHY M. Stress management classes as a health promotion tool. A Canadian Nurse, June 1981, pp. 29–31.

MYERS MF. Doctors' marriages. Plenum Press, New York, 1988:34.

NADELSON C, NOTMAN M. The woman physician. J Med Educ 1972; 47:176–184.

NEUWIRTH ZE. The silent anguish of the healers: patients suffer when physicians fall prey to stress. Newsweek, September 13, 1999, p. 79.

NIXON P. The human function curve: with special reference to: cardiovascular disorders. Practitioner 1976; 935:217,765,935.

PHELAN J, SCHWARTZ JE, BROMET EJ, et al. Work stress, family stress and depression in professional and managerial employees. Psych Med 1991; 21:999–1012.

POTTER RL. Resident, woman, wife, mother: issues for women in training. J Am Med Wom Assoc 1983; 38:4.

RAJ SR, SIMPSON CS, HOPMAN WM, SINGER MA. Health-related quality of life among final-year medical students. Can Med Assoc J 2000; 162:509–510.

REGELSON W. Physician "burnout." In: Wessels DT Jr, Kutscher AH, Seelang IB, et al, eds., Professional burnout in medicine and the helping professions. Haworth Press, New York, 1989. p 39–49.

RUBIN R, ORRIS P, LAU SL, HRYHORCZUK DO, FURNER S, LETZ R. Neurobehavioral effects of the on-call experience in housestaff physicians. J Occup Med 1991; 33:13–18.

SANDSON J. Moonlighting medical students. N Engl J Med 1985; 312:864.

SCHNALL PL, SCHWARTZ JE, LANDSBERGIS PA, WARREN K, PICKERING TG. A longitudinal study of job strain and ambulatory blood pressure: results from a three-year follow-up. Psychosom Med 1998; 60:697–706.

SCOTT N. The balancing act. Universal Press Syndicate, Kansas City, 1978.

SELDER FE, PAUSTIAN A. Burnout: absence of vision. In: Wessels DT Jr, Kutscher AH, Seelang IB, et al, eds. Professional burnout in medicine and the helping professions. Haworth Press, New York, 1989.

SELYE H. The stress of life. McGraw-Hill, New York, 1976.

SPEARS B. A time management system for preventing physician impairment. J Fam Pract 1981; 13:175–180.

SPIEGEL K, LEPROULT R, VAN CAUTER E. Impact of sleep debt on metabolic and endocrine function. Lancet 1999; 354:1435–1439.

TOEWS JA, LOCKYER JM, DOBSON DJG, et al. Analysis of stress levels among medical students, residents and graduate students at four Canadian schools of medicine. Acad Med 1997; 72:997–1002.

WALIS C. Stress—can we cope? Time, June 6, 1983, pg 63.

WOODS SM, NATTERSON J, SILVERMAN J. Medical students' disease: hypochondriasis in medical education. J Med Educ 1966; 41:785–790.

# CHAPTER 3

BARNETT RC, BEINER L, BARUCH GY, eds. Gender and stress. The Free Press, Macmillan, New York, 1987.

BELLE D. Gender differences in the social moderators of stress. In: Barnett RC, Beiner L, Baruch GY, eds. Gender and stress. The Free Press, Macmillan, New York, 1987: 257–277.

BLAKE RL, VANDIVER TA. The association of health with stressful life changes, social supports and coping. Fam Pract Res J 1988; 7(4):205–218.

BROWN M, SAKAI J, et al. A retraining program for inactive physicians. West J Med 1969; November:396–399.

BRUNTON SM, OSTERGAARD D. Report on a workshop on maternity and paternity leave held at the Directors of Family Practice Residency Program workshop, 1982. American Academy of Family Physicians, Leawood, Kansas.

CARTWRIGHT LIC, Role montage: life patterns of professional women. J Am Med Wom Assoc 1987; 42(5):142–148.

CLEARY PD. Gender differences in stress-related disorders. In: Barnett RC, Beiner L, Baruch GT, eds. Gender and stress. The Free Press, Macmillan, New York, 1987: 39–72.

CRAIGIE FC, LIU IY, LARSON DB, LYONS JS. A systematic analysis of religious variables in the *Journal of Family Practice* 1976–1986. J Fam Prac 1988; 27(5):509–513.

DAVIDSON V. Coping styles of women medical students. J Med Educ 1978; 53:902–907.

DOWLING C. The Cinderella complex. Simon and Schuster, New York, 1981.

GERBER L. Married to their careers. Tavistock, New York, 1983.

GLABMAN M. Coaching. Am Med News, January 5, 1998, pp. 13–14.

GOLISZEK A. 60 second stress management. New Horizons Press, Far Hills, New Jersey, 1992.

HEINS M, SMACK S, MARTINDALE L, et al. Comparison of productivity of women and men physicians. JAMA 1977; 237(23):2514–2517.

HOFERIK M, SARNOWSKI S. Feelings of loneliness in medical students. J Med Educ 1981; 56:397–403.

HOLMES PH, RAHLE RH. Social Readjustment Rating Scale. J Psychosom Res 1976; 11:216.

JASMINE S, HILL L, et al. The art of managing stress. Nursing, June 1981:53–57.

KAHN N, SCHAEFFER H. A process group approach to stress reduction and personal growth in a family practice residency program. J Fam Pract 1981; 12(6):1043–1047.

KING M, STANLEY G, BURROWS G. Stress: theory and practice Gram & Stratton, Orlando, FL, 1987.

KONANC J. What support groups for women medical students do: a retrospective inquiry. J Am Med Wom Assoc 1979; 34:282.

LAMBERG L. Roots of physician stress explored. JAMA 1999; 282(1):13–14.

LOEHR J. Stress for success. Random House, Toronto, Canada, 1997.

MCLEAN A. Work stress. Addison-Wesley, Reading MA, 1982: 277–299.

MURPHY M. Stress management classes as a health promotion tool. A Canadian Nurse June 1981: 29–31.

POST DM. Values, stress, and coping among practicing family physicians. Arch Fam Med 1997; 6:252–255.

RAPOPORT R, RAPOPORT R. Further considerations of a dual-career family. Hum Relat 1971; 24(6):519–533.

SHAPIRO E, DRISCOLI S. Part-time residencies versus shared scheduling. Resident and Staff Physician 1978; December:66–71.

SHAPIRO E, DRISCOLI S. Shared schedule training: compliance with section 709, P.L. 94-484. J Med Educ 1979; 54:576–578.

SHAPIRO E, LANE M, et al. The supply of reduced schedule residencies. J Am Med Wom Assoc 1980; 35(2):175–180.

SPEARS B. A time management system for prevention physician impairment. J Fam Pract 1981; 13:175–180.

SYMONDS A. The wife as the professional. Am J Psychoanal 1979; 39(1):552–563.

VOELKER R. MD's fear laws may limit home offices. Am Med News, May 26, 1989, pp. 15–17.

WALIS C. Stress—can we cope? Time, June 6, 1983, pg 63.

WETHINGTON E, MCLEOD JD, KESSLER RC. The importance of life events for explaining sex differences in psychological distress. In: Barnett RC, Beiner L, Baruch GY, eds. Gender and stress. The Free Press, Macmillan, New York, 1987: 144–156.

WINEBERG E. Retraining physicians. J Med Educ 1972; 47:625–630.

## CHAPTER 4

American Medical Association. Women in medicine in America: in the mainstream. American Medical Association, Chicago, 1991.

ANGELL M. Juggling a personal and professional life. J Am Med Wom Assoc 1982; 37(3):64–68.

BARNETT RC, BIENER L, BARUCH GK, eds. Gender and stress. The Free Press, Macmillan, New York, 1987.

BELLE D. Gender differences in the social moderators of stress. In: Barnett RC, Beiner L, Baruch GK, eds. Gender and stress. The Free Press, Macmillan, New York, 1987: 257–277.

CARTWRIGHT L. Career satisfaction and role harmony in a sample of young woman physicians. J Vocation Behav 1978; 12:184–196.

CLEARY PD. Gender differences in stress-related disorders. In: Barnett RC, Beiner L, Baruch GK, eds. Gender and stress. The Free Press, Macmillan, New York, 1987: 39–72.

DRALLE PW. Women physicians' name choices at marriage. J Am Med Wom Assoc 1987; 42(6):173–175.

EISENBERG L. Dystaff of Asculapius—the married woman as physician. J Am Med Wom Assoc 1981; 36(2):84–88.

FINE C. Married to medicine: an intimate portrait of doctors' wives. Atheneum, New York, 1981.

FRANK E, HARVEY L, ELON L. Family responsibilities and domestic activities of U.S. women physicians. Arch Fam Med 2000; 9:134–140.

GABBARD GO, MENNINGER W, eds. Medical marriages. American Psychiatric Press, Washington, DC, 1988.

GABBARD GO, MENNINGER RW. The psychology of postponement in the medical marriage. JAMA 1989; 261(16):2378–2381.

GERBER LA. Married to their careers. Tavistock, New York, 1983.

HEINS M. Medicine and motherhood. JAMA 1982; 249(2):209–210.

JOHNSON F, KAPLAN E, TUSEL D. Sexual dysfunction in the two-career family. Med Aspects Hum Sexuality 1979; 13(9):7–17.

KAPLAN H. Women physicians—the more effective recruitment and utilization of their talents and their resistance to it. Wom Physician 1970; 25(9):561–570.

LORBER J. How physicians' spouses influence each other's careers. J Am Med Wom Assoc 1982; 37(1):21–26.

McKAY MB, ALBOSZTA M, BINGCANG CC, et al. A stressor unique to married female physicians. Letter to the editor. Am J Psychiatry 1986; 143:114.

MYERS MF. Overview: female physician and her marriage. Am J Psychiatry 1984; 141:1386–1391.

MYERS MF. Doctors' marriages: a look at the problems and their solutions. Plenum, New York, 1988.

NADELSON CC, EISENBERG L. Successful professional women: on being married to one. Am J Psychiatry 1977; 134:10.

NADELSON CC, NOTMAN MT, LOWENSEIN P. The practice patterns, life styles, and stresses of women and men entering medicine: a follow-up study of Harvard medical school graduates from 1967 to 1977. J Am Med Wom Assoc 1979; 34(11):400–406.

NOTMAN MT, NADELSON CC. Psychological issues for the woman physician. In: Gabbard GO, Menninger RW, eds. Medical marriages. American Psychiatric Press, Washington DC 1988: 67–88.

OGLE KS, HENRY RC, DURDA K, ZIVICK JD. Gender-specific differences in family practice graduates. J Fam Pract 1986; 23(4):357–360.

PARKER G, JONES R. The doctor's husband. Br J Med Psychiatry 1981; 54:143–147.

POTTER RL. Resident, woman, wife, mother: issues for women in training. J Am Med Wom Assoc 1983; 38(4):98–102.

RAPOPORT R, RAPOPORT R. Further considerations on a dual-career family. Hum Relat 1971; 24(6):519–533.

ROLLMAN BL, MEAD LA, WANG N-Y, KLAG MJ. Medical specialty and the incidence of divorce. N Engl J Med 1997; 336(11):800–803.

SCHEIER R. Patterns set in residency persist throughout marriage. Am Med News, May 6, 1988, p. 31.

SCOTT N. The balancing act. Universal Press Syndicate, Kansas City, 1978.

SOBECKS NW, JUSTICE AC, HINZE S, et al. When doctors marry doctors: a survey exploring the professional and family lives of young physicians. Ann Intern Med 1999; 130:312–319.

SOTILE WM, SOTILE MO. The medical marriage: sustaining healthy relationships for physicians and their families, rev. ed. American Medical Association, Chicago, 2000.

SPENDLOVE DC, REED BD, WHITMAN N, et al. Marital adjustment among housestaff and new attorneys. Acad Med 1990; 65:599–603.

TESCH BJ, OSBORNE J, SIMPSON DE, MURRAY SF, SPIRO J. Women physicians in dual-physician relationships compared with those in other dual-career relationships. Acad Med 1992; 67:542–544.

THOMPSON M. The professional name of women physicians: a plea for constancy. New Physician, April, 1980, pp. 4–6.

VINCENT MO. Female physicians as psychiatric patients. Can Psych Assoc J 1976; 21(7):461–465.

WARDE C, ALLEN W, GELBERG L. Physician role conflict and resulting career changes: gender and generational differences. J Gen Intern Med 1996; 11:729–735.

WARDE CM, MOONESINGHE K, ALLEN W, GELBERG L. Marital and parental satisfaction of married physicians with children. J Gen Intern Med 1999; 14:157–165.

WETHINGTON E, MCLEOD JD, KESSLER RC. The importance of life events for explaining sex differences in psychological distress. In: Barnett RC, Beiner L, Baruch GK, eds. Gender and stress. The Free Press, Macmillan, New York, 1987: 144–156.

WINTER R. Course helps future M.D.'s balance career, family life. Am Med News, March 11, 1983, p. 26.

## CHAPTER 5

American Medical Association. Women in medicine in America: in the mainstream. AMA, Chicago, 1991.

American Medical Association. Women in medicine: 1998 data source. AMA, Chicago, 1998.

ANESHENSEL CS, PEARLIN LI. Structural contexts of sex differences in stress. In: Barnett RC, Beiner L, Baruch GK, eds. Gender and stress. The Free Press, Macmillan, New York, 1987. p 75–95.

ANGELL M. Juggling a personal and professional life. J Am Med Wom Assoc 1982; 37(3):64–68.

BARNETT RC, BIENER L, BARUCH GK, eds. Gender and stress. The Free Press, Macmillan, New York, 1987.

BIRD CE. Gender, household labor, and psychological distress: the impact of the amount and division of housework. J Health Soc Behav 1999; 40:32–45.

BONAR J, WATSON J, et al. Sex differences in career and family plans of medical students. J Am Med Wom Assoc 1982;37(11):300–303.

BROWN JB. Female family doctors: their work and well-being. Fam Med 1992; 24:591–595.

BRYANT HE, JENNETT PA, KISHINEVSKY M. Gender, family status, and career patterns of graduates of the University of Calgary Faculty of Medicine. Acad Med 1991; 66:483–485.

CARTWRIGHT L. Career satisfaction and role harmony in a sample of young women physicians. J Vocation Behav 1978; 12:184–196.

COHEN M, WOODWARD CA, FERRIER BM. Factors influencing career development: do men and women differ? J Am Med Wom Assoc 1988; 43(5):142–154.

EISENBERG L. Dystaff of Asculapius—the married woman as physician. J Am Med Wom Assoc 1981; 36(2):84–88.

FRANK E, HARVEY L. Family responsibilities and domestic activities of U.S. women physicians. Arch Fam Med 2000; 9:134–140.

GROSS EB. Gender differences in physician stress. J Am Med Wom Assoc 1992; 47:107–114.

HEINS M. Medicine and motherhood. JAMA 1982; 249(2):209–210.

HEINS M, SMOCK S, MARTINDALE L, et al. Comparison of productivity of women and men physicians. JAMA 1977; 237(23):2514–2517.

HOJAT M, GONNELLA JS, XU G. Gender comparisons of young physicians' perceptions of their medical education, professional life, and practice: a follow-up study of Jefferson Medical College graduates. Acad Med 1995; 70:305–312.

KAPLAN H. Women physicians—the more effective recruitment and utilization of their talents and their resistance to it. Wom Physician 1970; 25(9):561–570.

LORBER J. How physicians' spouses influence each other's careers. J Am Med Women Assoc 1982; 37(1):21–26.

NADELSON CC, EISENBERG L. Successful professional women: on being married to one. Am J Psychiatry 1977; 134:10.

NOCK SL, KINGSTON PL. Time with children: the impact of couples' work-time commitments. Soc Forces 1988; 67:59–85.

PFEIFFER RF. Early adult development in the medical student. Mayo Clin Proc 1983; 58:127–134.

RAPOPORT R, RAPOPORT R. Further considerations of a dual career family. Hum Relat 1971; 24(6):519–533.

SCHWARTZBERG NS, DYTELL RS. Dual-earner families: the importance of work stress and family stress for psychological well-being. J Occup Health Psych 1996; 1(2):211–223.

SHELTON BA. Women, men, and time: gender differences in paid work, housework, and leisure. Greenwood Press, New York, 1992.

SULLIVAN O. Time waits for no (wo)man: an investigation of the gendered experience of domestic time. Sociology 1997; 31:221–239.

TESCH BJ, OSBORNE J, SIMPSON DE, MURRAY SF, SPIRO J. Women physicians in dual-physician relationships compared with those in other dual-career relationships. Acad Med 1992; 67:542–544.

UHLENBERG P, COONEY TM. Male and female physicians: family and career comparisons. Soc Sci Med 1990; 30:373–378.

WARDE C, ALLEN W, GELBERG L. Physician role conflict and resulting career changes. J Gen Intern Med 1996; 11:729–735.

WOODWARD CA, WILLIAMS AP, FERRIER B, COHE M. Time spent on professional activities and unwaged domestic work: is it different for male and female primary care physicians who have children at home? Can Fam Physician 1996; 42:1938–1935.

## CHAPTER 6

American Medical Association. Women in medicine in America: in the mainstream. American Medical Association, Chicago, 1991.

BAUCOM-COPELAND S, COPELAND ET, PERRYLL. The pregnant resident: career conflict. J Am Med Wom Assoc 1983; 38(4):103–105.

BLUESTONE N. Marriage and medicine. J Am Med Wom Assoc 1965; 20(11):1048–1053.

CARR PL, ASH AS, FRIEDMAN RH, et al. Relation of family responsibilities and gender to productivity and career satisfaction of medical faculty. Ann Intern Med 1998; 129:532–538.

CASPER LM. What does it cost to mind our preschoolers? In: Current population reports. Census Bureau, P70-52, Washington, DC, September 1995.

FISH LS, NEW RS, VAN CLEAVE NJ. Shared parenting in dual-income families. Am J Orthopsychiatry 1992; 62(1):83–92.

FRANK E, CONE K. Characteristics of pregnant vs. non-pregnant women physicians: findings from the Women Physicians' Health Study. Int J Gynecol Obstet 2000; 69:37–46.

FRANK E, McMURRAY J, LINZER M, ELON L, Society of General Medicine Career Satisfaction Study Group. Career satisfaction of U.S. women physicians: results from the Women Physicians' Health Study. Arch Intern Med 1999; 159:1417–1426.

FRANK E, ROTHENBERG R, BROWN WV, MAIBACH H. Basic demographic and professional characteristics of US women physicians. West J Med 1997; 166:179–184.

FRIEDMAN R, BIGGER T, KORNFELD D. The intern and sleep loss. N Engl J Med 1971; 285(4):201–203.

GREENBAUM A, MINKOFF H, BLADE D. Pregnancy among obstetricians: a comparison of births before, during and after residency. Am J Obstet Gynecol 1987; 157:79–84.

GRISSO JA, HANSEN L, ZELLING I, BICKEL J, EISENBERG JM. Parental leave policies for faculty in U.S. medical schools. Ann Intern Med 1991; 114:43–45.

KAPLAN H. Women physicians—the more effective recruitment and utilization of their talents and their resistance to it. Wom Physician 1970; 25(9):561–570.

KLEBANOFF MA, SHIONO PH, RHOADS GG. Outcomes of pregnancy in a national sample of resident physicians. N Engl J Med 1990; 323:1040–1045.

ORDWAY J. Professional women's unanticipated contented feelings after the birth of a child. J Am Med Wom Assoc 1980; 35(10):240–245.

OSBORN LM, HARRIS DL, READING JC, PRATHER MB. Outcomes of pregnancies experienced during residency. J Fam Pract 1990; 6(31):618–622.

PFEIFFER RJ. Early adult development in the medical student. Mayo Clin Proc 1983; 58:127–134.

PHELAN ST. Pregnancy during residency: II. Obstetric complications. Obstet Gynecol 1988; 72(3):431–436.

POTTER RL. Resident, woman, wife, mother: issues for women in training. J Am Med Wom Assoc 1983; 38(4):103–105.

SAYRES M, WYSHAK G, DENTERLEIN G. Pregnancy during residency. N Engl J Med 1986; 314(7):418–423.

SCOTT N. The balancing act. Universal Press Syndicate, Kansas City, 1978.

SINAL S, WEAVIL P, CAMP MG. Survey of women physicians on issues relating to pregnancy during a medical career. J Med Educ 1988; 63:531–538.

SOBECKS NW, JUSTICE AC, HINZE S, et al. When doctors marry doctors: a survey exploring the professional and family lives of young physicians. Ann Intern Med 1999; 130:312–319.

STEIN BA, LEVENTHAL SE. Psychopathology in adolescent children of physicians. Can Med Assoc J 1984; 130:599–602.

STEPHEN B. What's the best time to have a baby? Redbook, February 1983, p. 36.

TESCH BJ, OSBORNE J, SIMPSON DE, MURRAY SF, SPIRO J. Women physicians in dual-physician relationships compared with those in other dual career relationships. Acad Med 1992; 7:542–544.

WARDE CM, MOONESINGHE K, ALLEN W, GELBERG L. Marital and parental satisfaction of married physicians with children. J Gen Intern Med 1999; 14:157–165.

WASSERMAN RC, HASSUK BM, YOUNG PC, LAND ML. Health care of physicians' children. Pediatrics 1989; 83(3):319–322.

ZYLKE JW. Among latchkey children problems: insufficient day-care facilities, data on possible harm. JAMA 1988; 260(23):3399–3400.

ZYLKE JW. Day-care quality and quantity become challenges for parents, politicians, and medical researchers. JAMA 1988; 260(22):3247–3249.

## CHAPTER 7

ACKERMAN-ROSS FS, SOCHAT N. Close encounters of the medical kind: attitudes toward male and female physicians. Soc Sci Med 1980; 14A:61–64.

BALDWIN DC, JR, DAUGHERTY SR, ECKENFELS EJ. Student perceptions of mistreatment and harassment during medical school—a survey of ten United States schools. West J Med 1991; 155:140–145.

BENSING JM, VAN DEN BRINK-MUINEN A, DE BAKKER DH. Gender differences in practice style: a Dutch study of general practitioners. Med Care 1993; 31:219–229.

BICKEL J, RUFFIN A. Gender-associated differences in matriculating and graduating medical students. Acad Med 1995; 70:551–559.

BROGAN DJ, FRANK E, ELON L, SIVANESAN SP, O'HANLAN KA. Harassment of lesbians as medical students and physicians. JAMA 1999; 282:1290,1292.

BUTLER D, GEIS FL. Nonverbal affect responses to male and female leaders: implications for leadership evaluations. J Pers Soc Psychol 1990; 58:48–59.

CARR PL, ASH AS, FRIEDMAN RH, et al. Faculty perceptions of gender discrimination and sexual harassment in academic medicine. Ann Intern Med 2000; 132:889–896.

CHALLACOMBE CB. Do women patients need women doctors? The Practitioner 1983; 227:848–850.

CONLEY FK. Toward a more perfect world—eliminating sexual discrimination in academic medicine. N Engl J Med 1993; 328:351–352.

COOK DJ, LIUTKUS JF, RISDON CL, et al. Residents' experiences of abuse, discrimination and sexual harassment during residency training. Can Med Assoc J 1996; 154: 1657–1665.

DRUZIN P, SHRIER I, YACOWAR M, ROSSIGNOL M. Discrimination against gay, lesbian and bisexual family physicians by patients. Can Med Assoc J 1998; 158:593–597.

ELNICKI DM, LINGER B, ASCH E, et al. Patterns of medical student abuse during the internal medicine clerkship: perspectives of students at 11 medical schools. Acad Med 1999; 74(S):S99–101.

ENGLEMAN EG. Attitudes toward women physicians. A study of 500 clinic patients. West J Med 1974; 120:95–100.

FRANK E, BROGAN D, SCHIFFMAN M. Prevalence and correlates of harassment among US women physicians. Arch Intern Med 1998; 158:352–358.

GARTRELL NK, MILLIKEN N, GOODSON WH III, THIEMANN S, LO B. Physician-patient sexual contact—prevalence and problems. West J Med 1992; 157:139–143.

HAAR E, HALITSKY V, STRICKER G. Factors related to the preference for a female gynecologist. Med Care 1975; 13(9):782–790.

HARTZEMA AG, CHRISTENSEN DB. Nonmedical factors associated with the prescribing volume among family practitioners in an HMO. Med Care 1983; 21(10):990–1000.

KASTELER JM, HUMLE S. Attitudes toward women physicians in a Mormon community. J Am Med Wom Assoc 1980; 35(2):37–41.

KOMAROMY M, BINDMAN AB, HABER RJ, SANDE MA. Sexual harassment in medical training. N Engl J Med 1993; 328:322–326.

LENHART SA, KLEIN F, FALCAO P, PHELAN E, SMITH K. Gender bias against and sexual harassment of AMWA members in massachusetts. J Am Med Wom Assoc 1991; 46:121–125.

LUBITZ RM, NGUYEN DD. Medical students abuse during third-year clerkships. JAMA 1996; 275:414–416.

NEEDLE RH, MURRAY BA. The relationship between race and sex of health provider, the quality of care provided, and levels of satisfaction with gynecological care among black college women. Coll Health, December 16, 1977, pp. 127–131.

PETRAVAGE JB, REYNOLDS LJ, GARDNER HJ, READING JC. Attitudes of women toward the gynecologic examination. J Fam Pract 1979; 9(6):1039–1045.

PHILLIBER SG, JONES J. Staffing a contraceptive service for adolescents: the importance of sex, race, and age. Public Health Rep 1982; 97(2):165–169.

PHILLIPS S, SCHNEIDER M. Sexual harassment of female doctors by patients. N Engl J Med 1993; 329:1936–1939.

REED SE. Our loss: the wage gap's huge cost. Ladies' Home Journal, August 1999, p. 62.

RICHMAN JA, FLAHERTY JA, ROSPENDA KM, CHRISTENSEN ML. Mental health consequences and correlates of reported medical student abuse. JAMA 1992; 267: 692–694.

ROSS CE, MIROWSKI J, DUFF RS. Physician status characteristics and client satisfaction in two types of medical practice. J Health Soc Behav 1982; 23:317–329.

SCHIFFMAN M, FRANK E. Harassment of women physicians. J Am Med Wom Assoc 1995; 46:121–125.

SCHNEIDER M, PHILLIPS SP. A qualitative study of sexual harassment of female doctors by patients. Soc Sci Med 1997; 45:669–676.

VAN NESS CJ, LYNCH DA. Male adolescents and physician sex preference. Arch Pediatr Adolesc Med 2000; 154:49–53.

WEYRAUCH KF, BOIKO PE, ALVIN B. Patient sex role and preference for a male or female physician. J Fam Pract 1990; 30:559–562.

## CHAPTER 8

ANDES GM. Mark Twain's cat. Ann Intern Med 1998; 128:1043–1044.

CALKINS DR, RUBENSTEIN LV, CLEARY PD, et al. Failure of physicians to recognize functional disability in ambulatory patients. Ann Intern Med 1991; 114:451–454.

IEZZONI LI. What should I say? Communication around disability [on being a patient]. Ann Intern Med 1998; 129:661–665.

IEZZONI LI. When walking fails [the patient-physician relationship]. JAMA 1996; 276:1609–1613.

IEZZONI LI, MCCARTHY EP, DAVIS RB, SIEBENS H. Mobility impairments and use of screening and preventive services. Am J Public Health 2000; 90:955–961.

MCNEIL JM. Americans with disabilities: data from survey of income and program participation. United States Census Bureau, Washington, DC, 1992.

NOSEK MA, HOWLAND CA. Breast and cervical cancer screening among women with physical disabilities. Arch Phys Med Rehabil 1997; 78:S39–44.

POPE AM, TARLOV AR. Disability in America: toward a national agenda for prevention. National Academy Press, Washington, DC, 1991.

PRICE R. A whole new life: an illness and a healing. Plume, New York, 1995.

RABIN D, RABIN PL, RABIN R. Compounding the ordeal of ALS: isolation from my fellow physicians. N Engl J Med 1982; 307:506–509.

Robert Wood Johnson foundation. Chronic Care in America: A 21st century challenge. http://www.chronicnet.org Princeton NJ 2001.

STETTEN D JR. Coping with blindness. N Engl J Med 1981; 305:458–460.

WAINAPEL SF. A clash of cultures: reflections of a physician with a disability. Lancet 1999; 254:763–764.

*www.wemedia.com*. This site is maintained by the publishers of *We* magazine, a consumer monthly magazine designed for people with disabilities.

ZOLA IK. Missing pieces: a chronicle of living with a disability. Temple University Press, Philadelphia, 1982.

## CHAPTER 9

American Medical Association Council on Scientific Affairs. Physician mortality and suicide: results and implication of the AMA-APA Physician Mortality Project, Stage II. American Medical Association, Chicago, 1986.

BALDWIN G, FRANK E, FIELDING B. Radon-related practices of U.S. women physicians. Am J Prev Med 1998; 15:49–53.

BLAZER DG, KESSLER RC, McGONAGLE KA, SWARTZ MS. The prevalence and distribution of major depression in a national community sample: The National Comorbidity Survey. Am J Psychiatry 1994; 151:979–986.

BOWMAN MA, ALLEN DI. Stress and women physicians, 2nd ed. Springer-Verlag, New York, 1990.

BROWN JB. Female family doctors: their work and well-being. Fam Med 1992; 24:591–595.

CRAIG AG, PITTS FN, JR. Suicide by physicians. Dis Nerv Syst 1968; 29:763–772.

DOYLE J, FRANK E, SALTZMAN LE, McMAHON PM, FIELDING BD. Domestic violence and sexual abuse in women physicians: associated medical, psychiatric, and professional difficulties. J Women's Health 1999; 8:955–965.

FIRTH-COZENS J. Source of stress in women junior house officers. BMJ 1990; 301: 89–91.

FRANK E, BHAT-SCHELBERT K, ELON L. Exercise counseling and personal exercise habits of U.S. women physicians. Under review.

FRANK E, BIOLA H, BURNETT CA. Mortality rates and causes among U.S. physicians. Am J Prev Med 2000; 19:155–159.

FRANK E, BROGAN DJ, MOKDAD AH, SIMOES EJ, KAHN HS, GREENBERG RS. Health-related behaviors of women physicians vs other women in the United States. Arch Intern Med 1998; 158:342–348.

FRANK E, DINGLE AD. Depression and suicide attempts among U.S. women physicians. Am J Psychiatry 1999; 156:1887–1894.

FRANK E, ROTHENBERG R, LEWIS C, BELODOFF B. Correlates of physicians' prevention-related practices: findings from the Women Physicians Health Study. Arch Fam Med 2000; 9:359–367.

HENDRIE HC, CLAIR DK, BRITTAIN HM, FADUL PE. A study of anxiety/depressive symptoms of medical students, house staff, and their spouses/partners. J Nerv Ment Dis 1990; 178:204–207.

HOLMES VF, RICH CL. Suicide among physicians. In: Blumenthal SJ, Dupfer DJ, eds. Suicide over the life cycle: risk factors, assessment, and treatment of suicidal patients. American Psychiatry Press, Washington, DC, 1990: 599–618.

HUGHES PH, BRANDENBURG N, BALDWIN DC JR, STORR CL, WILLIAMS KM, Sheehan DV: Prevalence of substance use among US physicians [published erratum appears in JAMA 1992;268:2518]. JAMA 1992; 267:2333–2339.

JOHNSTON C. Suicide totals for MDs safe reminder of stresses facing medicine, conference told. Can Med Assoc J 1996; 155:109–111.

KEMM J. Alcohol and heart disease: the implications of the U-shaped curve [editorial]. BMJ 1993; 307:1373–1374.

LaRosa JH. Executive women and health: perceptions and practices. Am J Public Health 1990; 80:1450–1454.

LIBERATOS P, LINK BG, KELSEY JL. The measurement of social class in epidemiology [review]. Epidemiol Rev 1988; 10:87–121.

LINDEMANN S, LAARA E, HAKKO H, LONNQVIST J. A systematic review on gender specific mortality in medical doctors. Br J Psychiatry 1996; 168:274–279.

MCNAGNY SE, WENGER NK, FRANK E. Personal use of postmenopausal hormone replacement therapy by women physicians in the United States. Ann Intern Med 1997; 127:1093–1096.

MOSCICKI EK, O'CARROLL A, RAE DS, LOCKE BZ, ROY A, REGIER DA. Suicide attempts in the Epidemiologic Catchment Area study. Yale J Biol Med 1988; 61:259–268.

OLKINUORA M, ASP S, JUNTUNEN J, KAUTTU K, STRID L, AARIMAA M. Stress symptoms, burnout, and suicidal thoughts in Finnish physicians. Soc Psychiatry Psychiatr Epidemiol 1990; 25:81–86.

PITTS FN JR, SCHULLER AB, RICH CL, PITTS AF. Suicide among US women physicians, 1967. Am J Psychiatry 1979; 136:694–696.

RICH CL, PITTS FN JR. Suicide by male physicians during a five-year period. Am J Psychiatry 1979; 136:1089–1090.

ROSE KD, ROSCOW I. Physicians who kill themselves. Arch Gen Psychiatry 1973; 29:800–805.

ROY A. Suicide in doctors. Psychiatr Clin North Am 1985; 8:377–387.

STAMPFER MJ, COLDITZ GA, WILLETT WC, SPEIZER FE, HENNEKENS CH. A prospective study of moderate alcohol consumption and the risk of coronary disease and stroke in women. N Engl J Med 1988; 319:267–273.

STEPPACHER R, MAUSER JS. Suicide in male and female physicians. JAMA 1974; 228:323–328.

THOMAS CB. What becomes of medical students: the dark side. Johns Hopkins Med J 1976; 130:105–195.

ULLMANN D, PHILLIPS RL, BEESON L, et al. Cause-specific mortality among physicians with differing life-styles. JAMA 1991; 265:2352–2359.

VON BRAUCHITCH H. The physicians' suicide revisited. J Med Dis 1976; 162:40–45.

WATTERSON DJ. Pyschiatric illness in the medical profession—incidence in relation to sex and field of practice. Can Med Assoc J 1976; 115:311–317.

WELLS KB, LEWIS CE, LEAKE B, WARE JE JR. Do physicians preach what they practice? A study of physicians' health habits and counseling practices. JAMA 1984; 252:3846–3848.

WINKLEBY MA, JATULIS DE, FRANK E, FORMANN SP. Socioeconomic status and health: how education, income, and occupation contribute to risk factors for cardiovascular disease. Am J Public Health 1992; 82:816–820.

WYSHAK G, LAMB GA, LAWRENCE RS, CURRAN WJ. A profile of the health-promoting behaviors of physicians and lawyers. N Engl J Med 1980; 303:104–107.

## CHAPTER 10

AAMC. Report of the AAMC Task Force to the Inter-Association Committee on Expanding Education Opportunities in Medicine for Blacks and Other Minority Students. Association of American Medical Colleges, Washington, DC, 1970.

AAMC. Statistical information. Faculty in US medical schools. Association of American Medical Colleges, Washington, DC, 2000.

AAMC. Statistical information related to medical education. Facts: applicants and matriculants and graduates. Association of American Medical Colleges, Washington, DC, 1998.

AMARO H, RUSSO NF, et al. Family and work predictors of psychological well-being among Hispanic women professionals. Psychol Wom Q 1987; 11(4):505–521.

BALDWIN D JR, DAUGHERTY S, et al. Racial and ethnic discrimination during residency: results of a national survey. Acad Med 1994; 69(10 suppl):S19–S21.

BLACKWELL J. Mentoring: an action strategy for increasing minority faculty. Academe 1982; 75:8–14.

BONNETT A, DOUGLAS F. Black medical students in white medical schools. Social Policy 1983; 14:23–26.

CARLISLE D, GARDNER J, et al. The entry of underrepresented minority students in US medical schools: an evaluation of recent trends. Am J Public Health 1998; 88(9):1314–1318.

COHEN A, CANTOR J, et al. Young physicians and the medical profession. Health Affairs 1990; 9:138–148.

CORBIE-SMITH G, FRANK E, et al. The intersection of race, gender and primary care: results from the Women Physicians' Health Study. J Natl Med Assoc 2000; 92:472–480.

CORBIE-SMITH G, FRANK E, et al. Prevalences and correlates of ethnic harassment in the US Women Physicians' Health Study. Acad Med 1999; 74(6):695–701.

DAVIDSON R, LEWIS E. Affirmative action and other special consideration admissions at the University of California, Davis, School of Medicine. JAMA 1997; 278(14): 1153–1158.

HADLEY J, CANTOR JC, et al. Young physicians most and least likely to have second thoughts about a career in medicine. Acad Med 1992; 67(3):180–190.

HANFT RS, WHITE CC. Constraining the supply of physicians: effects on black physicians. Milbank Q 1987; 65(suppl 2):249–269.

JACKSON JS, BROWN TN, et al. Racism and the physical and mental health status of African-Americans: a thirteen year national panel study. Ethnicity Dis 1996; 6(1–2): 132–147.

JOHNSON DG, LLOYD SM, et al. A second survey of graduates of a traditionally black college of medicine. Acad Med 1989; 64(2):87–94.

KEITH SN, BELL RM, et al. Affirmative action in medical education and its effect on Howard and Meharry: a study of the class of 1975. J Natl Med Assoc 1988; 80(3):153–158.

KEITH SN, BELL RM, et al. Effects of affirmative action in medical schools: a study of the class of 1975. N Engl J Med 1985; 313:1519–1525.

LAVIZZO-MOUREY R, CLAYTON LA, et al. The perceptions of African-American physicians concerning their treatment by managed care organizations. J Natl Med Assoc 1996; 88(4):210–214.

LEVINSON W, WEINER J. Promotion and tenure of women and minorities on medical school faculties. Ann Intern Med 1991; (114):63–68.

MENGES R, EXUM WH. Barriers to the progress of women and minority faculty. J Higher Educ 1983; 54:123–144.

MOY E, BARTMAN B. Physician race and care of minority and medically indigent patients. JAMA 1995; 273:1515–1520.

MURPHY JM, NADELSON CC, et al. Factors influencing first-year medical students' perceptions of stress. J Hum Stress 1984; 10(4):165–173.

NICKENS H, READY T, et al. Project 3000 by 2000: racial and ethnic diversity in U.S. Medical schools. N Engl J Med 1994; 331(7):472–476.

PALEPU A, CARR P, et al. Minority faculty and academic rank in medicine. JAMA 1998; 280(9):767–771.

PETERSDORF R, TURNER K, et al. Minorities in medicine: past, present and future. Acad Med 1990; 65(11):663–670.

The Pew Health Professions Commission. Recreating health professionals practice for a new century. 1998.

READY T, NICKENS HW. Black men in the medical education pipeline: past, present, and future. Acad Med 1991; 66(4):181–187.

SHEEHAN K, SHEEHAN D, et al. A pilot study of medical student abuse. Student perceptions of mistreatment and misconduct in medical chool. JAMA 1990; 263(4): 533–537.

SHERVINGTON D, BLAND I, et al. Ethnicity, gender identity, stress, and coping among female African-American medical students. J Am Med Wom Assoc 1996; 51(4): 153–154.

SIMPSON CE JR, ARONOFF R. Factors affecting the supply of minority physicians in 2000. Public Health Rep 1998; 103(2):178–184.

SUINN RM, WITT JC. Survey on ethnic minority faculty recruitment and retention. Am Psychology 1982; 37:1239–1244.

U.S. Census Bureau. Population projections of the United States by age, sex, race, and Hispanic origin: 1995 to 2050. In: Current population reports. U.S. Census Burean, Washington, DC, 1998.

WHITCOMB M. Correcting the oversupply of specialist by limiting residencies for graduates of foreign medical schools. N Engl J Med 1995; 333(7):454–456.

WILSON D, KACZMAREK J. The history of African-American physicians and medicine in the United States. J Assoc Acad Minority Phys 1993 (3):93–98.

## CHAPTER 11

American College of Sports Medicine. Guidelines for exercise testing and prescription. Lea and Febiger, Philadelphia, 1986.

BACHMAN R, SALTZMAN LE. Violence against women: estimates from the redesigned survey. Bureau of Justice Statistics Special Report. US Department of Justice, Washington, DC;1995.

BALDWIN G, FRANK E, FIELDING B. Radon-related practices of U.S. women physicians. Am J Prev Med 1998; 15:49–53.

BLAZER DG, KESSLER RC, MCGONAGLE KA, SWARTZ MS. The prevalence and distribution of major depression in a national community sample: the National Comorbidity Survey. Am J Psychiatry 1994; 151:979–986.

CHAN B, ANDERSON G, THERIAULT M. Patterns of practice among older physicians in Ontario. Can Med Assoc J 1998; 159:1101–1106.

CORBIE-SMITH G, FRANK E, NICKENS II, ELON L. Prevalence and correlates of ethnically-based harassment in U.S. women physicians. Acad Med 1999; 74:695–701.

DeFRIES Z. Identity matters (or does it?) JAMA 1998; 279:1331.

DOYLE J, FRANK E, SALTZMAN LE, McMAHON PM, FIELDING BD. Domestic violence and sexual abuse in women physicians: associated medical, psychiatric, and professional difficulties. J Wom Health 1999; 8:955–965.

FRANK E. Political self-characterization of U.S. women physicians. Soc Sci Med 1999; 48:1475–1481.

FRANK E, BENDICH A, DENNISTON M. Use of vitamin/mineral supplements by U.S. women physicians. Am J Clin Nutr, 2000; 72:969–975.

FRANK E, BROGAN D, MOKDAD AH, SIMOES E, KAHN H, GREENBERG RS. Health-related behaviors of women physicians vs other women in the United States. Arch Intern Med 1998a; 158:342–348.

FRANK E, BROGAN D, SCHIFFMAN M. Harassment experiences of U.S. women physicians. Arch Intern Med 1998b; 158:352–358.

FRANK E, DELL ML, CHOPP R. Religious characteristics of U.S. women physicians. Soc Sci Med 1999a; 49:1717–1722.

FRANK E, DINGLE AD. Depression and suicide attempts among U.S. women physicians. Am J Psychiatry 1999; 156:1887–1894.

FRANK E, FEINGLASS S. Student loan debt does not predict specialty choice among US women physicians. J Gen Intern Med 1999; 14:347–350.

FRANK E, HARVEY L. Family responsibilities and domestic activities of U.S. women physicians. Arch Fam Med 2000; 9:134–140.

FRANK E, KELLERMAN A. Gun ownership in U.S. women physicians. South Med J 1999; 92:1083–1088.

FRANK E, MCMURRAY J, LINZER M, ELON L, Society of General Medicine Career Satisfaction Study Group. Career satisfaction of U.S. women physicians: results from the Women Physicians' Health Study. Arch Intern Med 1999b; 159:1417–1426.

FRANK E, ROTHENBERG R, BROWN V, MAIBACH H. Basic demographic and professional characteristics of U.S. women physicians. West J Med 1997; 166:179–184.

FRANK E, ROTHENBERG R, LEWIS C, FIELDING B. Correlates of physicians' prevention-related practices: findings from the Women Physicians' Health Study. Arch Fam Med 2000; 75:359–367.

HALL GH. Medicine to serve and aging society: retired doctors could have a role. BMJ 2000; 320:7232.

KOSS MP. Hidden rape: sexual aggression and victimization in a national sample of students in higher education. In: Burgess AW, ed. Rape and sexual assault, vol 2. Garland New York, 1988: 3–25.

ROBB N. Interest in physician-buyout packages grows as more doctors contemplate retirement. Can Med Assoc J 1997; 156:882–888.

Technical support document for the 1992 citizen's guide to radon. EPA publication no. 400-R-92-011. U.S. Environmental Protection Agency, Office of Radiation Programs, Radon Division, Washington, DC, 1992.

## CHAPTER 12

AAMC Project Committee on Increasing Women's Leadership in Academic Medicine. Executive summary. Acad Med 1996; 71:801–811.

American College of Physicians. Promotion and tenure of women and minorities on medical school faculties. Ann Intern Med 1991; 114:63–68.

BENZ E, CLAYTON CP, COSTA ST. Increasing academic internal medicine's investment in female faculty. Am J Med 1998; 105:459–463.

BICKEL J, CROFT K, MARSHALL R. Women in U.S. academic medicine statistics 1998. Association of American Medical Colleges, Washington, DC, 1998.

BLAND CJ, SCHMITZ CC. Characteristics of the successful researcher and implications for faculty development. J Med Educ 1986; 61:22–31.

BRASLOW JB, HEINS M. Women in medical education: a decade of change. N Engl J Med 1981; 304:1129–1135.

BRIGHT CM, DUEFIELD CA, STONE VE. Perceived barriers and biases in the medical education experience by gender and race. J Natl Med Assoc 1998; 90:681–688.

CALKINS EV, ARNOLD LM, WILLOUGHBY TL. Gender differences in predictors of performance in medical training. J Med Educ 1987; 62:682–685.

CARR PL, ASH AS, FRIEDMAN RH, et al. Relation of family responsibilities and gender to the productivity and career satisfaction of medical faculty. Ann Intern Med 1998; 12:532–538.

CARR PL, FRIEDMAN RH, MOSKOWITZ MA, KAZIS LE. Comparing the status of women and men in academic medicine. Ann Intern Med 1993; 119:908–913.

CARR P, FRIEDMAN RH, MOSKOWITZ MA, KAZIS LE, WEED HG. Research, academic rank, and compensation of women and men faculty in academic general internal medicine. J Gen Intern Med 1992; 7:418–432.

CASE SM, BECKER DF, SWANSON DB. Performances of mend and women on NBME Part I and Part II: the more things change . . . Acad Med 1993; 68:S25–S27.

CASE SM, HATALA R, BLAKE J, GOLDEN GS. Does sex make a difference? Sometimes it does and sometimes it doesn't. Acad Med 1999; 74:S37–S40.

CASE SM, SWANSON DB, RIPKEY DR, et al. Performance of the class of 1994 in the new era of USMLE. Acad Med 1996; 71:S91–S93.

CROVITZ E. Women entering medical school: the challenge continues. J Am Med Wom Assoc 1980; 35(12):291–298.

DAWSON B, IWAMOTO CK, ROSS LP, et al. Performance on the National Board of Medical Examiners part I examination by men and women of different race and ethnicity. JAMA 1994; 272:674–679.

DAY SC, NORCINI JJ, SHEA JA, BENSON JA JR. Gender differences in the clinical competence of residents in internal medicine. J Gen Intern Med 1989; 4:309–312.

EAGLY A et al. Gender and the effectiveness of leaders: a meta-analysis. Psychol Bull 1995; 117:125–145.

FIORENTINE R. Men, women, and the premed persistence gap: a normative alternatives approach. Am J Soc 1987; 92(5):1118–1139.

HEALY B. Women in science: from panes to ceilings. Science 1992; 255:1333.

HEID IM, O'FALLON JR, SCHWENK NM, GABRIEL SE. Increasing the proportion of women in academic medicine: one institution's response. Mayo Clin Proc 1999; 74:113–119.

HERMAN MW, VELOSKI JJ. Premedical training, personal characteristics and performance in medical school. Med Educ 1981; 15:363–367.

HUFF KL, FANG D. When are students most at risk of encountering academic difficulty? A study of 1992 matriculants to U.S. Medical Schools. Academic Medicine 1999; 74:454–460.

JOHNSON DG. US medical students 1950–2000. Association of American Medical Colleges, Washington DC, 1983.

KWAKWA F, JONASSON O. Attrition in graduate surgical education: an analysis of the 1993 entering cohort of surgical residents. J Am Coll Surg 1999; 189:602–610.

LEVINSON W, KAUFMAN K, CLARK B, TOLLE SW. Mentors and role models for women in academic medicine. West J Med 1991; 154:423–426.

LEVINSON W, TOLLE SW, LEWIS C. Women in academic medicine: combining career and family. N Engl J Med 1989; 321:1511–1517.

MARQUART JA, FRANCO KN, CARROLL BT. The influence of applicants' gender on medical school interviews. Acad Med 1990; 65:410–411.

MATTHEWS MR. The training and practice of women physicians: a case study. J Med Educ 1970; 45:1016–1024.

MENDELSOHN KD, NIEMAN LZ, ISAACS K, LEE S, LEVISON SP. Sex and gender bias in anatomy and physical diagnosis text illustrations. JAMA 1994; 272:1267–1270.

NICKERSON KG, BENNETT NM, ESTES D, SHEA S. The status of women at one academic medical center. JAMA 1990; 264:1813–1817.

NONNEMAKER L. Women physicians in academic medicine: new insights from cohort studies. N Engl J Med 2000; 342:399–405.

NORCINI JJ, FLETCHER SW, QUIMBY BB, SHEA JA. Performance of women candidates on the American Board of Internal Medicine certifying examination, 1973–1982. *Ann Intern Med* 1985; 102:115–118.

OGGINS J, INGLEHART M, BROWN DR, MOORE W. Gender differences in the prediction of medical students' clinical performance. J Am Med Wom Assoc 1988; 43(6):171–175.

PINN VW. Commentary: women, research and the National Institutes of Health. Am J Prev Med 1992; 8:324–327.

RAND VE, HUDES ES, BROWNER WS, WACHTER RM, AVINS AL. Effect of evaluator and resident gender on the American Board of Internal Medicine Evaluation Scores. J Gen Intern Med 1998; 13:670–674.

RUTALA PJ, WITZKE DB, LEKO EO, FULGINITI JV. Threats to the validity of scores on standardized patient examinations. Acad Med 1991; 66:S28–S30.

SOLOMON DJ, SPEER AJ, AINSWORTH MA, DIPETTE DJ. Investigating gender bias in preceptors' ratings of medical students. Acad Med 1993; 68:703.

TESCH BJ, WOOD HM, HELWIG AL, NATTINGER AB. Promotion of women physicians in academic medicine: glass ceiling or sticky floor? JAMA 1995; 273:1022–1025.

WILLOUGHBY L, CALKINS V, ARNOLD L. Different predictors of examination performance for male and female medical students. J Am Med Wom Assoc 1979; 34(8):316–320.

WOLLSTADT LJ, GRAVDAL J, GLASSER M. Gender and the educational experience in a primary care training setting. Fam Med 1990; 22:210–214.

## CHAPTER 13

BAKER LC. Differences in earnings between male and female physicians. N Engl J Med 1996; 334:960–964.

BATES AS, HARRIS LE, TIERNEY WM, WOLINSKY FD. Dimensions and correlates of physician work satisfaction in a Midwestern city. Med Care 1998; 36:610–617.

BEIL C, SICK DR, MILLER WE. A comparison of specialty choices among senior medical students using Bem sex-role inventory scale. J Am Med Wom Assoc 1980; 35(7): 178–181.

BOBULA JD. Work patterns, practice characteristics, and incomes of male and female physicians. J Med Educ 1980; 55:826–833.

BURNLEY CS, BURKETT GL. Specialization: are women in surgery different? J Am Med Wom Assoc 1986; 41(5):144–152.

CHAMBERS R, CAMPBELL I. Gender differences in general practitioners at work. Br J Gen Pract 1996; 46:291–293.

DUCKER DG. Believed suitability of medical specialties for women physicians. J Am Med Wom Assoc 1978; 33(1):25,29–32.

DYKMAN RA, STALNAKER JM. Survey of women physicians graduating from medical school in 1925–1940. J Med Educ 1957; 32:3–38.

ELLSBURY K, SCHNEEWEISS R, MONTANO DE, GORDON KC, KUYKENDALL D. Gender differences in practice characteristics of graduates of family medicine residencies. J Med Educ 1987; 62:895–903.

FRANK E, MCMURRAY J, LINZER M, ELON L, Society of General Medicine Career Satisfaction Study Group. Career satisfaction of U.S. women physicians: results from the Women Physicians' Health Study. Arch Intern Med 1999; 159:1417–1426.

FRANK E, ROTHENBERG R, BROWN WV, MAIBACH H. Basic demographic and professional characteristics of US women physicians. West J Med 1997; 166:179–184.

GOLDBLATT A, GOLDBLATT PB. The status of women physicians: a comparison of USMG, women, USMG men, and FMGs. J Am Med Wom Assoc 1976; 31(8):325–328.

GONZALEZ ML. Gender differences in physician earnings and practice patterns. *http://www.ama-assn.org/advocacy/healthpolicy/x-ama/gender.htm.* 1999.

HAAS JS, CLEARY PD, PUOPOLO AL, et al, and the Ambulatory Medicine Quality Improvement Project Investigators. Differences in the professional satisfaction of general internists in academically affiliated practices in the greater Boston area. J Gen Intern Med 1998; 13:127–130.

HEINS M, SMOCK S, MARTINDALE L, JACOBS J, STEIN M. Comparison of the productivity of women and men physicians. JAMA 1977; 237(23):2514–2517.

HOJAT M, GONNELLA JS, VELOSKI JJ, MOSES S. Differences in professional activities, perceptions of professional problems, and practice patterns between men and women graduates of Jefferson Medical College. Acad Med 1990; 65:755–761.

KROL D, MORRIS V, BETZ J, CADMAN E. Factors influencing the career choices of physicians trained at Yale–New Haven Hospital from 1929–1994. Acad Med 1998; 73(3):313–317.

LEE RH, MROZ TA. Family structure and physicians' hours in large, multispecialty groups. Inquiry 1991; 38:366–374.

MATTERA MD. Female doctors: why they're on an economic treadmill. Med Econ, February 18, 1980, pp. 98–101.

MITCHELL JB. Why do women physicians work fewer hours than men physicians? Inquiry 1984; 21:361–368.

MITKA M. Women doctor' liability premiums edging closer to men's. Am Med News, October 21, 1991, p. 14.

OGLE KS, HENRY RC, DURDA K, ZIVICK JD. Gender-specific differences in family practice graduates. J Fam Pract 1986; 23(4):357–360.

PASKO T, SEIDMAN B. Physician characteristics and distribution in the US. American Medical Association, Chicago, 1999.

SILBERGER AA, MARDER WD, WILLKE RJ. Practice characteristics of male and female physicians. Health Affairs 1987;winter:104–109.

SLOAN FA, MERGENHAGEN PM, BURFIELD WB, et al. Medical malpractice experience of physicians: predictable or haphazard? JAMA 1989; 262(23):3291–3297.

SMITH RS. A profile of lawyer lifestyles. Am Bar Assoc J 1984; 70:50.

STAMPS PL, PIEDMONTE EB, HAASE AB, SLAVITT DB. Measurement of work satisfaction among health professionals. Med Care 1978; 16:337–352.

# CHAPTER 14

BADGER LW, BERBAUM M, CARNEY PA, DIETRICH AJ, et al. Physician-patient gender and the recognition and treatment of depression in primary care. J Social Serv Res 1999; 25:21–39.

BELENKY MF, CLINCHY BMcV, GOLDBERGER NR, TARULE JM. Women's ways of knowing. Basic Books, New York, 1986.

BENSING JM, VAN DEN BRINK-MUINEN A, DE BAKKER DH. Gender differences in practice style: a Dutch study of general practitioners. Med Care 1993; 31:219–229.

BERGQUIST SR, DUCHAC BW, SCHALIN VA, et al. Perceptions of freshman medical students of gender differences in medical specialty choice. J Med Educ 1985; 60: 379–383.

BERNZWEIG J, TAKAYAMA JI, PHIBBS C, et al. Gender differences in physician-patient communication—evidence from pediatric visits. Arch Pediatr Adolesc Med 1997; 151:586–591.

BEST DL, WILLIAMS JE, BRIGGS SR. A further analysis of the affective meanings associated with male and female sex-trait stereotypes. Sex Roles 1980; 6(5):735–746.

BOUCHARD L, RENAUD M. Female and male physicians' attitudes toward prenatal diagnosis: a pan-Canadian survey. Soc Sci Med 1997; 44(3):381–392.

BRITT H, BHASALE A, MILES DA, et al. The sex of the general practitioner—a comparison of characteristics, patients, and medical conditions managed. Med Care 1996; 34:403–415.

BROVERMAN IK, BROVERMAN DM, CLARKSON FE, ROSENKRANTZ PS, VOGEL SR. Sex-role stereotypes and clinical judgments of mental health. J Consult Clin Psychol 1970; 34(1):1–7.

BROVERMAN IK, VOGEL SR, BROVERMAN DM, CLARKSON FE, ROSENKRANTZ PS. Sex-role stereotypes: a current appraisal. J Soc Issues 1972; 28(2):59–78.

BUTLER D, GEIS FL. Nonverbal affect responses to male and female leaders: implications for leadership evaluations. J Pers Soc Psychol 1990; 58:48–59.

CARTWRIGHT LK. Personality differences in male and female medical students. Psychiatry Med 1972; 3:213–218.

CHAMBERS R, CAMPBELL I. Gender differences in general practitioners at work. Br J Gen Pract 1996; 46:291–293.

CLARK DC, ZELDOW PB. Vicissitudes of depressed mood during four years of medical school. JAMA 1988; 260(17):2521–2528.

COPLIN JW, WILLIAMS JE. Women law students' descriptions of self and the ideal lawyer. Psychol Women Q 1978; 2(4):323–333.

COULTER A, PETO V, DOLL H. Influence of sex of general practitioner on management of menorrhagia. Br J Gen Pract 1995; 45:471–475.

CROWSON TW, RICH EC, HARRIS IB. A comparison of locus of control between men and women in an internal medicine residency. J Med Educ 1986; 61:840–841.

DAVIS SW, BEST DL, MARION G, WALL GH. Sex stereotypes in the self- and ideal descriptions of physician's assistant student. J Med Educ 1984; 59:678–680.

DEAUX K, EMSWILLER T. Explanations of successful performance on sex-linked tasks: what is skill for the male is luck for the female. J Pers Soc Psychol 1974; 29(1): 80–85.

DEAUX K, WHITE L, FARRIS E. Skills versus luck: field and laboratory studies of male and female preferences. J Pers Soc Psychol 1975; 32(4):629–636.

DICKINSON GE, PEARSON AA. Sex differences of physicians in relating to dying patients. J Am Med Wom Assoc 1979; 34:45–47.

ELLSBURY K, SCHNEEWEISS R, MONTANO DE, GORDON KC, KUYKENDALL D. Gender differences in practice characteristics of graduates of family medicine residencies. J Med Educ 1987; 62:895–903.

ENGLEMAN EG. Attitudes toward women physicians. A study of 500 clinic patients. West J Med 1974; 120:95–100.

EWING GB, SELASSIE AW, LOPEZ CH, MCCUTCHEON FP. Self-report of delivery of clinical preventive services by US physicians—comparing specialty, gender, age, setting of practice, and area of practice. Am J Prev Med 1999; 17(1):62–72.

FEATHER NT. Attribution of responsibility and valence of success and failure in relation to initial confidence and task performance. J Pers Soc Psychol 1969; 13(2):129–144.

FEATHER NT, SIMON JG. Reactions to male and female success and failure in sex-linked occupations: impressions of personality, causal attributions, and perceived likelihood of different consequences. J Pers Soc Psychol 1975; 31(1):20–31.

FELDMAN-SUMMERS S, KIESLER SB. Those who are number two try harder: the effect of sex on attributions of causality. J Pers Soc Psychol 1974; 30(6):846–855.

FIORENTINE R. Men, women and the premed persistence gap: a normative alternatives approach. Am J Sociol 1987; 92(5):1118–1139.

FISHER H. Expert forecast: will women ever gain employment parity with men? The Wall Street Journal, January 1, 2000, p. R36.

FRANK E, HARVEY LK. Prevention advice rates of women and men physicians. Arch Fam Med 1996; 5:215–219.

FRANKS P, CLANCY CM. Physician gender bias in clinical decision making: screening for cancer in primary care. Med Care 1993; 31:213–218.

FREY J, DEMICK J, BIBACE R. Variations in physicians' feeling of control during a family practice residency. J Med Educ 1981; 56:50–56.

FRIEZE IH, WHITLEY BE, HANUSA BH, MCHUGH MC. Assessing the theoretical models for sex differences in causal attributions for success and failure. Sex Roles 1982; 8(4):333–343.

GILES H, WILLIAMS JE. Medical students' descriptions of self and ideal physician. Soc Sci Med 1979; 13A:813–815.

GILLIGAN C. In a different voice. Harvard University Press, Cambridge, MA, 1982.

GREER S, DICKERSON V, SCHNEIDERMAN LJ, et al. Responses of male and female physicians to medical complaints in male and female patients. J Fam Pract 1986; 23(1): 49–53.

GROSS W, CROVITZ E. A comparison of medical students' attitudes toward women and women medical students. J Med Educ 1975; 50:392–394.

HALL JA, IRISH JT, ROTER DL, EHRLICH CM, MILLER LH. Gender in medical encounters: an analysis of physician and patient communication in a primary care setting. Health Psychol 1994; 13:384–392.

HALL JA, PALMER RH, ORAV EJ, et al. Performance quality, gender and professional role—a study of physicians and nonphysicians in 16 ambulatory care practices. Med Care 1990; 28:489–501.

HARTZEMA AG, CHRISTENSEN DB. Nonmedical factors associated with the prescribing volume among family practitioners in an HMO. Med Care 1983; 21(10):990–1000.

HIGHLEN PS, GILLIS SF. Effects of situational factors, sex, and attitude on affective self-disclosure and anxiety. J Couns Psychol 1978; 25(4):270–276.

HOFFMAN DM, FIDELL LS. Characteristics of androgynous, undifferentiated, masculine, and feminine middle-class women. Sex Roles 1979; 5(6):765–781.

HOFFMAN LW. Early childhood experiences and women's achievement motives. J Social Issues 1972; 28(2):129–155.

HOJAT M, GONNELLA JS, XU G. Gender comparisons of young physicians' perceptions of their medical education, professional life and practice: a follow-up study of Jefferson medical college graduates. Acad Med 1995; 70:305–312.

JACKLIN CN. Methological issues in the study of sex-related differences. Dev Rev 1981; 1:266–273.

KREUTER MW, STRECHER VJ, HARRIS R, KOBRIN SC, SKINNER CS. Are patients of women physicians screened more aggressively? J Gen Intern Med 1995; 10:119–125.

LENNEY E. Women's self-confidence in achievement settings. Psychol Bull 1977; 84(1): 1–13.

LESERMAN J. Men and women in medical school: how they change and how they compare. Praeger, New York, 1981.

LEVINSON RM, McCOLLUM KT, KUTNER NG. Gender homophily in preferences for physicians. Sex Roles 1984; 19:315–325.

LEVY S, DOWLING P, BOULT L, et al. The effect of physician and patient gender on preventive medicine pracices in patients older than fifty. Fam Med 1992; 24(1):58–61.

LORBER J. Women physicians: careers, status, and power. Tavistock, New York, 1984.

LURIE N, MARGOLIS K, McGOVERN PG, MINK P. Physician self-report of comfort and skill in providing preventive care to patients of the opposite sex. Arch Fam Med 1998; 7(2):134–137.

LURIE N, MARGOLIS K, McGOVERN PG, MINK P, SLATER JS. Why do patients of female physicians have higher rates of breast and cervical cancer screening? J Gen Intern Med 1997; 12(1):34–43.

LURIE N, SLATER J, McGOVERN P, et al. Preventive care for women: does the sex of the physician really matter? N Engl J Med 1993; 329:478–482.

MAHEUX B, DUFORT F, BELAND F. Professional and sociopolitical attitudes of medical students: gender differences reconsidered. J Am Med Wom Assoc 1988; 43(3):73–76.

MAHEUX B, DUFORT F, BELAND F, JACQUES A, LEVESQUE A. Female medical practitioners: more preventive and patient oriented? Med Care 1990; 28:87–92.

MAJERONI BA, KARUZA J, WADE C, et al. Gender of physicians and patients and preventive care for community-based older adults. J Am Board Fam Pract 1993; 6: 359–365.

McGEE MG. Human spatial abilities: psychometric studies and environmental, genetic, hormonal, and neurological influences. Psychol Bull 1979; 86(5):889–918.

Medica. Women doctors sued less often. Medica 1983; winter:29–30.

MITKA M. Women doctor' liability premiums edging closer to men's. Am Med News October 21, 1991, p. 14.

National Ambulatory Medical Care Survey, United States, 1977. Characteristics of visits to female and male physicians. U.S. Department of Health and Human Services, Public Health Service, Office of Health Research, Statistics and Technology, National Center for Health Statistics. Publication no. (PHS) 80-1710, Hyattsville, MD, June 1980.

National Ambulatory Medical Care Survey, United States, January 1980a–December 1981a. Patterns of ambulatory care in general and family practice. U.S. Department of Health and Human Services, Public Health Service, National Center for Health Statistics. Publication no. (PHS) 83-1734, Hyattsville, MD, September 1983.

National Ambulatory Medical Care Survey, United States, January 1980b–December 1981b. Patterns of ambulatory care in pediatrics. U.S. Department of Health and Human Services, Public Health Service, National Center for Health Statistics. Publication no. (PHS) 84-1736, Hyattsville, MD, October 1983.

National Ambulatory Medical Care Survey, United States, January 1980c–December 1981c. Patterns of ambulatory care in obstetrics and gynecology. U.S. Department of Health and Human Services, Public Health Service, National Center for Health Statistics. Publication No. (PHS) 84-1737, Hyattsville, MD, February 1984.

OGLE KS, HENRY RC, DURDA K, ZIVICK JD. Gender-specific differences in family practice graduates. J Fam Pract 1986; 23(4):357–360.

RESTAK R. We need more cheap, docile women doctors. Washington Post, April 27, 1986. p C1, C4.

REZLER AG, BUCKLEY JM. A comparison of personality types among female student health professionals. J Med Educ 1977; 52:475–477.

RIESSMAN CK. Interview effects in psychiatric epidemiology: a study of medical and lay interviewers and their impact on reported symptoms. Am J Public Health 1979; 69(5):485–491.

ROESSLER R, COLLINS F, MEFFERD RB JR. Sex similarities in successful medical school applicants. J Am Med Wom Assoc 1975; 30(6):254–265.

ROTER D, LIPKIN M, KORSGAARD. Sex differences in patients' and physicians' communication during primary care medical visits. Med Care 1991; 29:1083–1093.

SCHUENEMAN AL, PICKLEMAN J, FREEARK RJ. Age, gender, lateral dominance, and prediction of operative skill among general surgery residents. Surgery 1985; 98(3): 506–513.

SETO TB, TAIRA DA, DAVIS RB, et al. Effect of physician gender on the prescription of estrogen replacement therapy. J Gen Intern Med 1996; 11:197–203.

SHAPIRO J, MCGRATH E, ANDERSON RC. Patients', medical students', and physicians' perceptions of male and female physicians. Percept Motor Skills 1983; 56:179–190.

SLOAN FA, MERGENHAGEN PM, BURFIELD WB, et al. Medical malpractice experience of physicians: predictable or haphazard? JAMA 1989; 262(23):3291–3297.

WEISMAN CS, NATHANSON CA, TEITELBAUM MA, CHASE GA, KING TM. Abortion attitudes and performance among male and female obstetrician-gynecologists. Fam Plann Perspect 1986; 18(2):67–73.

WEISMAN CS, NATHANSON CA, TEITELBAUM MA, CHASE GA, KING TM. Delivery of fertility control services by male and female obstetrician-gynecologists. Am J Obstet Gynecol 1987; 156:464–469.

WEISMAN CS, TEITELBAUM MA. Physician gender and the physician-patient relationship: recent evidence and relevant questions. Soc Sci Med 1985; 20(11):1119–1127.

WEST C. Reconceptualizing gender in physician-patient relationships. Soc Sci Med 1993; 36:57–66.

WILLIAMS JE, BEST DL. Sex stereotypes in education, occupation, and mental health. In: Williams JE, Best DL, eds. Measuring sex stereotypes: a thirty nation study. Sage, New York, 1982: 289–303.

WILLOUGHBY L, CALKINS V, ARNOLD L. Different predictors of examination performance for male and female medical students. J Am Med Wom Assoc 1979; 34(8): 316–320.

YOUNG JW. Symptom disclosure to male and female physicians: effects of sex, physical attractiveness, and symptom type. J Behav Med 1979; 2(2):159–169.

ZARE N, SORENSON JR, HEEREN T. Sex of provider as a variable in effective genetic counseling. Soc Sci Med 1984; 19(7):671–675.

# OTHER RESOURCES

## BOOKS

ABRAM R, Ed. Send us a lady physician: women doctors in American 1835–1920. W.W. Norton, New York, 1985.

American Medical Association. Women in Medicine in america: In the mainstream. American Medical Association, Chicago, 1995.

BICKER J, CLARK V, LAWSON R. Women in U.S. academic medicine statistics 1998–1999. Association of American Medical Colleges, Washington, DC, 1999.

CONLEY FK. Walking out on the boys. Farrar, Straus & Giroux, New York, 1998.

CORNELL V. The true story of a country physician in the Colorodo Rockies. Ballantyne, New York, 1991.

Council on Graduate Medical Education. Fifth Report. Publication no. HRSA-P-DM-95-1. Women and Medicine. Health Resources and Services Administration, US Department of Health and Human Services, Washington, DC, July 1995.

FURST LR, ed. Women healers and physicians. University Press of Kentucky, Lexington, KY, 1997.

GABBARD GO, MENNINGER RW, eds. Medical marriages. American Psychiatric Press, Washington, DC, 1988.

HADDAD AM, BROWN KH, Eds. The arduous touch: women's voices in health care. Purdue University Press, West Lafayette, IN, 1999.

KLASS P. Baby doctor: a pediatrician's training. Random House, New York, 1992.

KLASS P. A not entirely benign procedure: four years as a medical student. New American Library/Signet, New York, 1987.

KLASS P. Other women's children. Random House/Ivy, New York, 1992.

Ko K. The survival bible for women in medicine. Parthenon, Pearl River, NY, 1998.

Maines RP. The technology of orgasm: "hysteria," the vibrator, and women's sexual satisfaction. Johns Hopkins University Press, Baltimore, 1999.

More ES. Restoring the balance: women physicians and the profession of medicine, 1850–1995. Harvard University Press, Cambridge, MA, 1999.

More ES, Milligan MA, eds. The empathic practitioner: empathy, gender and medicine. Rutgers University Press, New Brunswick, NJ, 1994.

Pasko T, Seidman B. Physician characteristics and distribution in the US. American Medical Association, Chicago, 1999.

Pringle R. Sex and medicine. Cambridge University Press, Cambridge, UK, 1998.

Remen RN. Kitchen table wisdom. Riverhead, New York, 1996.

Salber EJ. The mind is not the heart. Duke University Press, Durham, NC, 1989.

Sotile WM, Sotile MO. Medical marriage: sustaining healthy relationships for physicians and their families rev. ed. American Medical Association, Chicago, 2000.

Toth E. Ms. Mentor's impeccable advice for women in academia. University of Pennsylvania Press, Philadelphia, 1997.

## WEB SITES/LISTSERVES

Please note Web sites and their addresses are subject to rapid change.

*SherifK@medcolpa.edu*—Where-L offers opportunities for networking and resource sharing for health care providers, educators, and students in the field of women's health.

*Vclark@aamc.org*—AAMC Women in Medicine (WIM) Listserve is a quick and easy way to share information with your colleagues. We invite you to share ideas for local WIM sponsored events, employment announcements, or *research questions* with over 100 members of the WIM listserve.

*Women-health@umich.edu*—U. of Michigan offers a guide to women's health issues that presents health issues of special concern to women.

*www.ama-assn.org*—American Medical Association for women.

*www.amsa.org*—American Medical Student Association.

*www.amwa-doc.org*—American Medical Woman's Association (AMWA) has a new electronic newsletter and a redesigned Web page featuring a new section called "advocacy," listing legislative priorities and agendas.

*www.astr.ua.edu/4000WS*—A database that lists the accomplishments of pre–20th century women in health and medicine. It is a good way togather information on our foremothers.

*www.medscape.com/Topics/WomensHealth/WomensHealth.mhtml*—Medscape, Inc. offers an online peer-reviewed journal, the first of its kind on women's health, with clinical news and full-text articles on a broad scope of women's health problems.

*www.4physicians.com*

*www.4women.gov/owh/pub/woc/index.htm*—The National Women's Health Information Center (new data book: Women of Color Health Data Book) is intended to help women health advocates and teachers understand the health status of women of color and assist them in addressing their needs.

*www.med.stanford.edu/school/facultymentoring*—Stanford University School of Medicine's Faculty Mentoring Program includes its history and guidelines for mentoring events, and other resources for faculty.

*http://research.med.umkc.edu/teams/cml/womendrs.html*—This site provides a listing of women physicians' autobiographies.

*http://endeavor.med.nyu.edu/lit-med/lit-med-db/webdocs/web keywords/women.in.medicine.kw.html*—This site provides literature related to medicine, with an emphasis on what the Web site developers feel would be of particular interest to women physicians. Each citation is annotated.

*www.residentpage.com*—American Hospital Association resident page.

## A SERIES OF WEB SITES OFFERING HELP TO PARENTS AND WOMEN

*www.IRS.ustreas.gov*—The IRS Web site where you can download all forms.

*www.familyboards.go.com*

*www.family.com*

*www.femalephysician.com*—A Web site designed specifically for female physicians.

*www.Ivillage.com*

*www.parentsplace.com*

*www.voiceofwomen.com*

*www.women.msn.com*

# BIBLIOGRAPHY FOR THE WOMEN PHYSICIANS' HEALTH STUDY*

## MAIN PAPERS

Frank E. 1995. "The Women Physicians Health Study: Background, Objectives and Methods." *Journal of the American Medical Women's Association.* Vol. 50, pgs. 64–66.

Frank E, Rothenberg R, Brown V, Maibach H. 1997. "Basic demographic and professional characteristics of US women physicians." *Western Journal of Medicine.* Vol. 166, pgs. 179–184.

Frank E, Brogan D, Mokdad AH, Simoes E, Kahn II, Greenberg RS. 1998. "Health-related behaviors of women physicians vs other women in the United States." *Archives of Internal Medicine.* Vol. 158, pgs. 342–348.

Frank E, Rothenberg R, Lewis C, Fielding B. 2000. "Correlates of physicians' prevention-related practices: findings from the Women Physicians' Health Study." *Archives of Family Medicine.* Vol 9, pgs. 359-367.

## SUBTOPICS

Schiffman M, Frank E. 1995. "Harassment of women physicians." *Journal of the American Medical Women's Association.* Vol. 50, pgs. 207–211.

McNagny S, Wenger N, Frank E. 1997. "Personal use of postmenopausal hormone replacement therapy by women physicians in the United States." *Annals of Internal Medicine.* Vol. 127, pgs. 1093–1096.

Frank E, Brogan D, Schiffman M. 1998. "Prevalence and correlates of harassment among US women physicians." *Archives of Internal Medicine.* Vol. 158, pgs. 352–358.

*For an updated bibliography, see http://med.emory.edu/WPHS/.

Baldwin G, Frank E, Fielding B. 1998. "U.S. women physicians' residential radon testing practices." *American Journal of Preventive Medicine*. Vol. 15, pgs. 49–53.

White R, Seymour J, Frank E. 1999. "Prevalence and effects of vegetarianism in U.S. women physicians." *Journal of the American Dietetic Association*. Vol. 99, pgs. 595–597.

Frank E. 1999. "Political self-characterization of U.S. women physicians." *Social Science and Medicine*. Vol. 48, pgs. 1475–1481.

Frank E, Hudgins P. 1999. "Academic vs. nonacademic women physicians: data from the Women Physicians' Health Study." *Academic Medicine*. Vol. 74, pgs. 553–556.

Frank E, Clancy C. 1999. "U.S. women physicians' assessment of the health care quality they receive." *Journal of Women's Health*. Vol. 8, pgs. 95–102.

Frank E, McMurray J, Linzer M, Elon L, Society of General Medicine Career Satisfaction Study Group. 1999. "Career Satisfaction of U.S. Women Physicians: Results from the Women Physicians' Health Study." *Archives of Internal Medicine*. Vol. 159, pgs. 1417–1426.

Brogan DJ, Frank E, Elon L, Sivaneson SP, O'Hanlan KA. 1999. "Harrassment of lesbians as medical students and physicians." *MS Journal of the American Medical Association*. Vol. 282, pgs. 1290–1292.

Corbie-Smith G, Frank E, Nickens H, Elon L. 1999. "Prevalences and correlates of ethnic harassment in U.S. women physicians." *Academic Medicine*. Vol. 74, pgs. 695–701.

Frank E, Feinglass S. 1999. "Student loan debt does not predict choosing a primary care specialty for US women physicians." *Journal of General Internal Medicine*. Vol. 14, pgs. 347–350.

Frank E, Kellerman A. 1999. "Firearm ownership among female physicians in the United States." *Southern Medical Journal*. Vol. 92, pgs. 1083–1088.

Frank E. 1999. "Contraceptive use by female physicians in the United States." *Obstetrics and Gynecology*. Vol. 94, pgs. 666–671.

Frank E, Dell ML, Chopp R. 1999. "Religious characteristics of U.S. women physicians." *Social Science and Medicine*. Vol. 49, pgs. 1717–1722.

Frank E, Dingle AD. 1999. "Self-reported depression and suicide attempts among U.S. women physicians." *American Journal of Psychiatry*. Vol. 156, pgs. 1887–1894.

Doyle J, Frank E, Saltzman LE, McMahon PM, Fielding BD. 1999. "Domestic violence and sexual abuse in women physicians: associated medical, psychiatric, and professional difficulties." *Journal of Women's Health*. Vol. 8, pgs. 955–965.

Frank E, Baldwin G, Langleib A. 2000. "Continuing medical education habits of U.S. women physicians." *Journal of the American Medical Women's Association*. Vol. 55, pgs. 27–28.

Frank E, Harvey L. 2000. "Family responsibilities and domestic activities of U.S. women physicians." *Archives of Family Medicine*. Vol. 9, pgs. 134–140.

Saraiya M, Frank E, Elon L, Baldwin G, McAlpine BE. 2000. "Personal and clinical skin cancer prevention practices of U.S. women physicians." *Archives of Dermatology*. Vol. 136, pgs. 633–642

Frank E, Cone K. 2000. "Characteristics of pregnant vs. nonpregnant women physicians: findings from the women physicians' health study." *International Journal of Gynecology and Obstetrics*. Vol. 69, pgs. 37–46.

Frank E, Sperling L, Wu K. 2000. "Aspirin use among women physicians in the United States." *American Journal of Cardiology*. Vol. 86, pgs. 465–466.

Frank E, Rimer BK, Brogan D, Elon L. 2000. "U.S. women physicians' personal and clinical breast cancer screening practices." *Journal of Women's Health*. Vol. 9, pgs. 791–801.

Frank E, Bendich A, Denniston M. 2000. "Use of vitamin-mineral supplements by female physicians in the United States." *American Journal of Clinical Nutrition.* Vol. 72, pgs. 969–75.

Corbie-Smith G, Frank E, Nickens H. 2000. "The intersection of race, gender, and primary care: results from the women physicians' health study." *Journal of the National Medical Association.* Vol. 92, pgs. 472–480.

Brogan D, Frank E, Elon L, O'Hanlan K. 2001. "Methodologic Concerns in Defining Lesbian for Health Research." *Epidemiology.* Vol. 12, pgs. 109–113.

Saraiya M, Coughlin S, Burke W, Elon L, Frank E. 2001. "The role of Family History in Personal and Clinical Cancer Prevention Practices among U.S. Women Physicians." *Community Genetics.* Vol. 4, pgs. 102–108.

Easton A, Husten C, Malarcher A, Elon L, Caraballo R, Ahluwalia I, Frank E. 2001. "Smoking cessation counseling by primary care women physicians: Women Physicians' Health Study." *Journal of Women's Health.* Vol. 32(4), pgs. 77–91.

Frank E, Wright E, Serdula M, Elon L, Baldwin G. 2001. "Personal and professional nutrition-related practices of US female physicians." *American Journal of Clinical Nutrition.* Vol. 75(2), pgs. 326–332.

Easton A, Husten C, Elon L, Frank E. "Specialist Physicians and Smoking Cessation Counseling: Women Physicians' Health Study." *Women and Health.* In press.

## STRATIFICATIONS BY SPECIALTY

Frank E, Brownstein M, Ephgrave L, Neumayer L. 1998. "Characteristics of women surgeons in the United States." *American Journal of Surgery.* Vol. 176, pgs. 244–250.

Frank E, Lutz L. 1999. "Characteristics of women US family physicians." *Archives of Family Medicine.* Vol. 8, pgs. 313–318.

Frank E, Vydareny K. 1999. "Characteristics of women radiologists in the United States." *American Journal of Roentgenology.* Vol. 173, pgs. 531–537.

Frank E, Rock J, Sara D. 1999. "Characteristics of Female Obstetrician-Gynecologists in the United States." *Obstetrics and Gynecology.* Vol. 94, pgs. 659–665.

Frank E, Totten V, Andrew L. 2000. "Characteristics of women emergency physicians." *Internet Journal of Emergency and Intensive Care Medicine.* Vol. 4.

Frank E, Meacham L. 2001. "Characteristics of US women pediatricians." *Clinical Pediatrics.* Vol. 40, pgs. 17–25.

Frank E, Boswell L, Dickstein L, Chapman D. 2001. "Characteristics of female psychiatrists." *American Journal of Psychiatry.* Vol. 158, pgs. 205–212.

Frank E, Singh S. 2001. "Personal and practice-related characteristics of a subsample of U.S. women dermatologists data from the Women Physicians' Health Study." *International Journal of Dermatology.* Vol 40(6), pgs. 393–400

Frank E, Kunovich-Frieze T, Corbie-Smith G. "Characteristincs of women internist." *Medscape General Medicine.* In press.

# INDEX